PLACEMENT OF EKG LEADS:

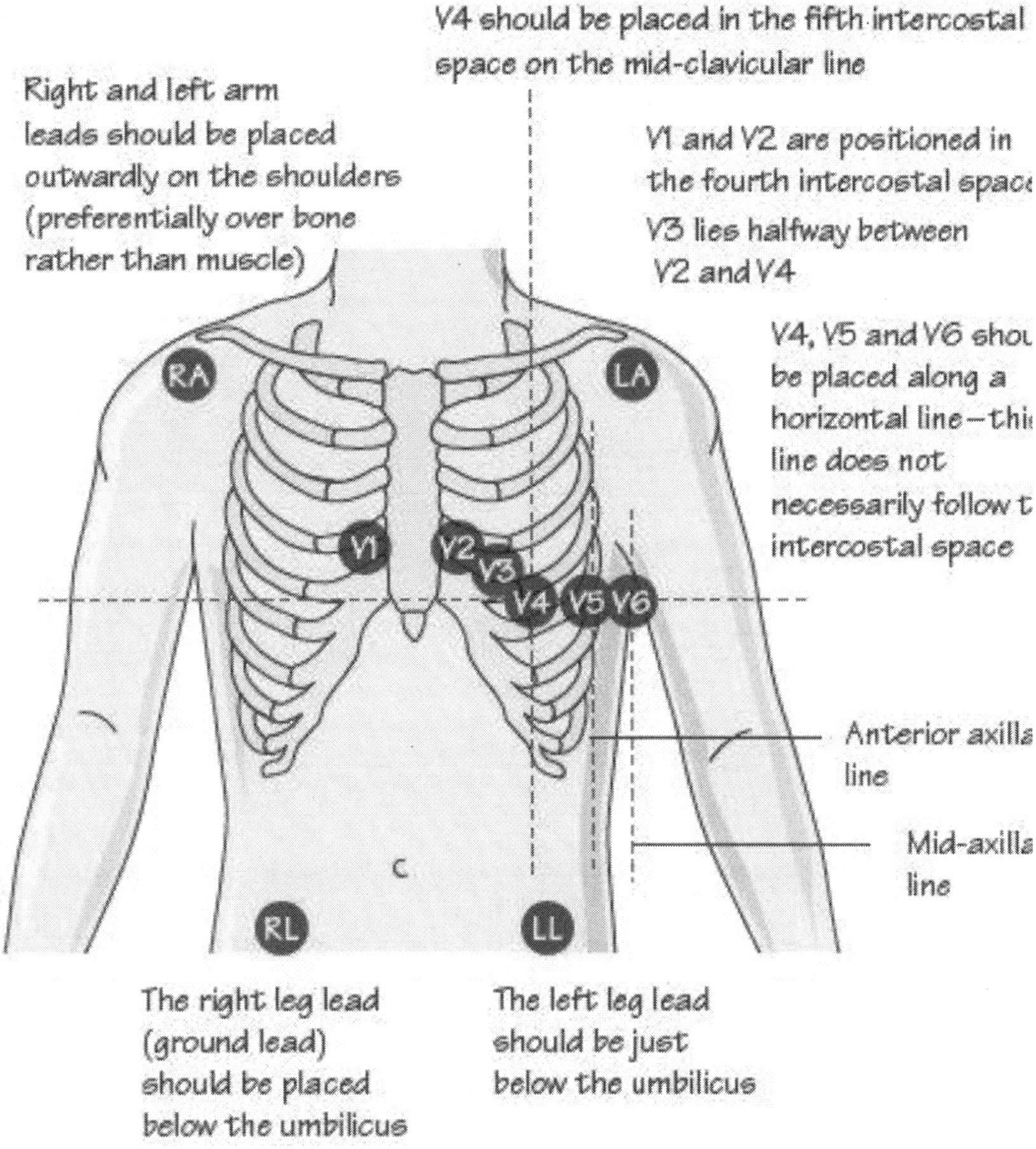
V4 should be placed in the fifth intercostal space on the mid-clavicular line
Right and left arm leads should be placed outwardly on the shoulders (preferentially over bone rather than muscle)
V1 and V2 are positioned in the fourth intercostal spac
V3 lies halfway between V2 and V4
V4, V5 and V6 shou be placed along a horizontal line—thi line does not necessarily follow t intercostal space
RA
LA
V1
V2
V3
V4
V5
V6
Anterior axilla line
Mid-axilla line
RL
LL
The right leg lead (ground lead) should be placed below the umbilicus
The left leg lead should be just below the umbilicus

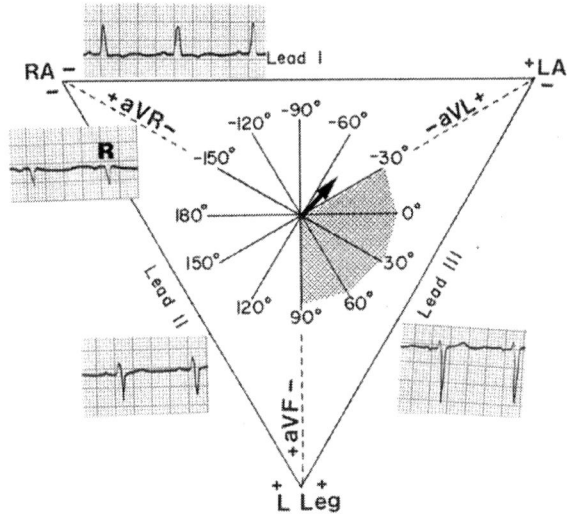

Learning to interpret 12 Lead EKG's does not have to be a daunting task. Some find the learning a painful and "head aching" venture. However once you understand the basic rules it is little more than repetition. In this book there are nearly 100 real 12 Lead EKG's. Take your time with each and you will be flying through 12 Leads in no time.

First:

A. Label the 12 Lead at how it identifies the section of the heart.

1. Lead I: High Lateral
2. Lead II: Inferior
3. Lead III: Inferior
4. AVR: Lead II mirror.
5. AVL: High Lateral
6. AVF: Inferior
7. V1: Septal

8. V2: Septal
9. V3: Anterior
10. V4: Anterior
11. V5: Low Lateral
12. V6: Low Lateral

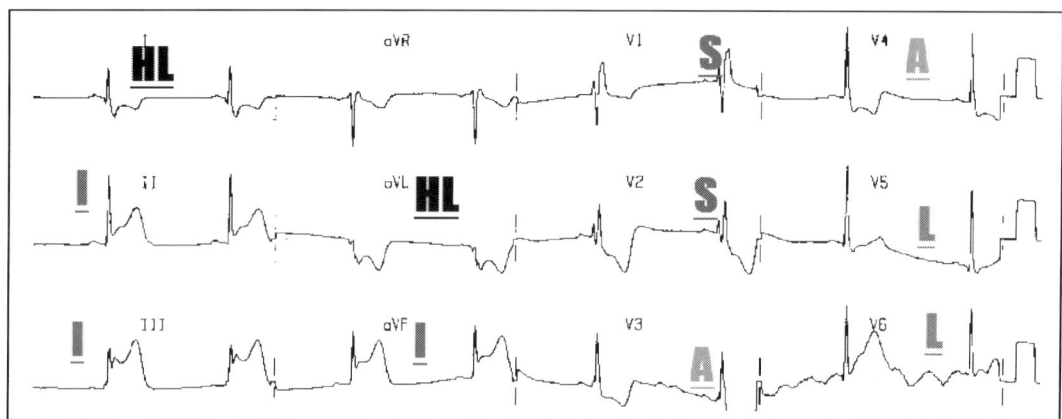

We have a memory aid to learn how to label the 12 Lead:

<u>A</u>ll Asses <u>I</u>n <u>I</u>raq <u>I</u>ncluding <u>L</u>ittle <u>H</u>abib are a <u>L</u>ittle <u>H</u>arry

When you start labeling the 12 Lead EKG go from right to left spelling out your memory aid. Oh...don't get offended by the memory aid, I came up with that while in Iraq with my Iraq counterparts who called me Habib...*they thought it was hilarious.*

Second:

B. Circle all signs of ectopy, elevation, ischemia, , or irregularities.

1. You don't have to circle everything if there is a lot but give yourself plenty examples.

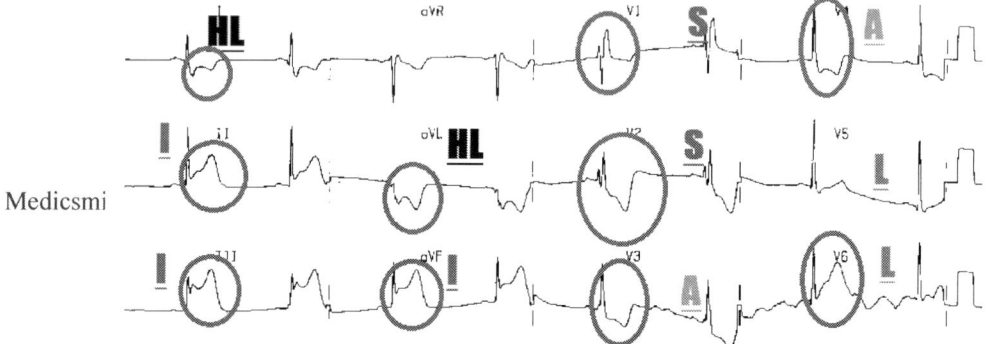

C. Write down the areas that you have circled from identified issues in the EKG.

1. "Q" waves must be at least 2/3 the size of the "RS" complexes to be considered an active MI.

2. Damage or ischemia must be shown in at least 2 contiguous leads to be an active MI.

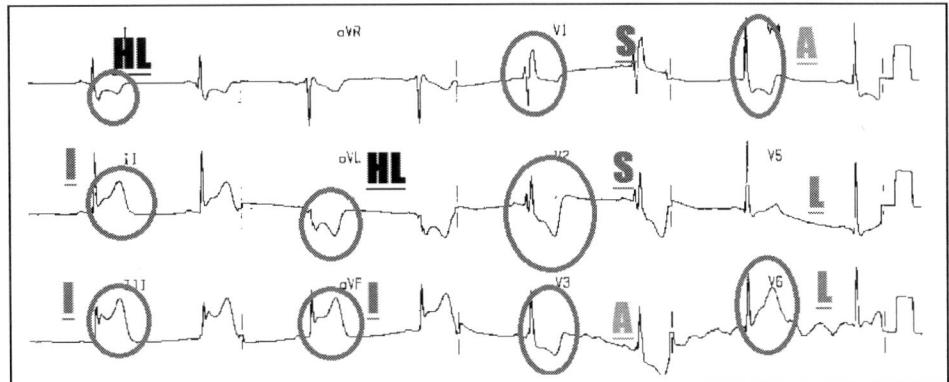

a. **Inferior ST elevation**

b. **High Lateral Ischemia**

c. **Septal Ischemia**

d. **Anterior Ischemia**

e. **Diagnosis: Inferior & Lateral Wall AMI**

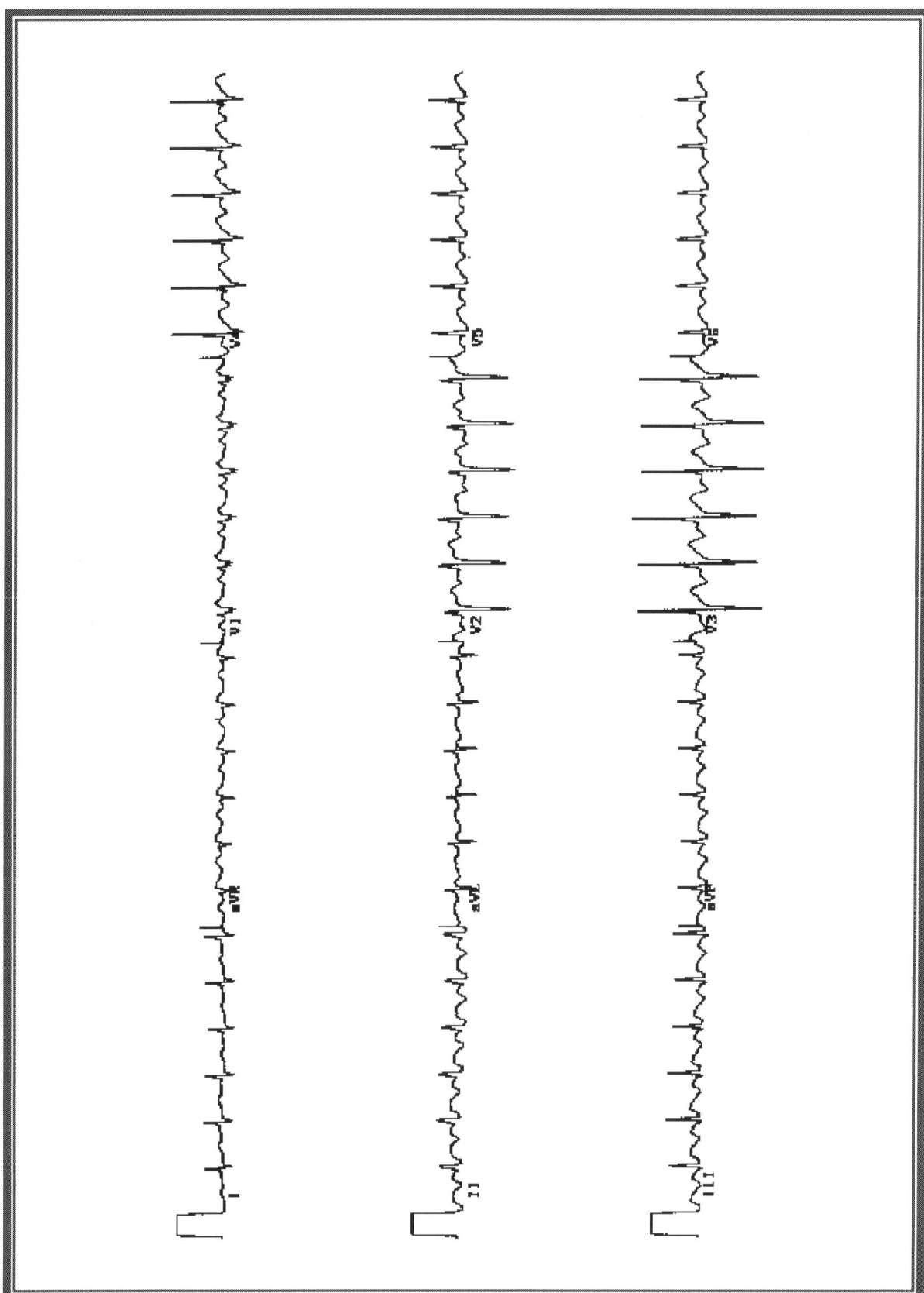

blank

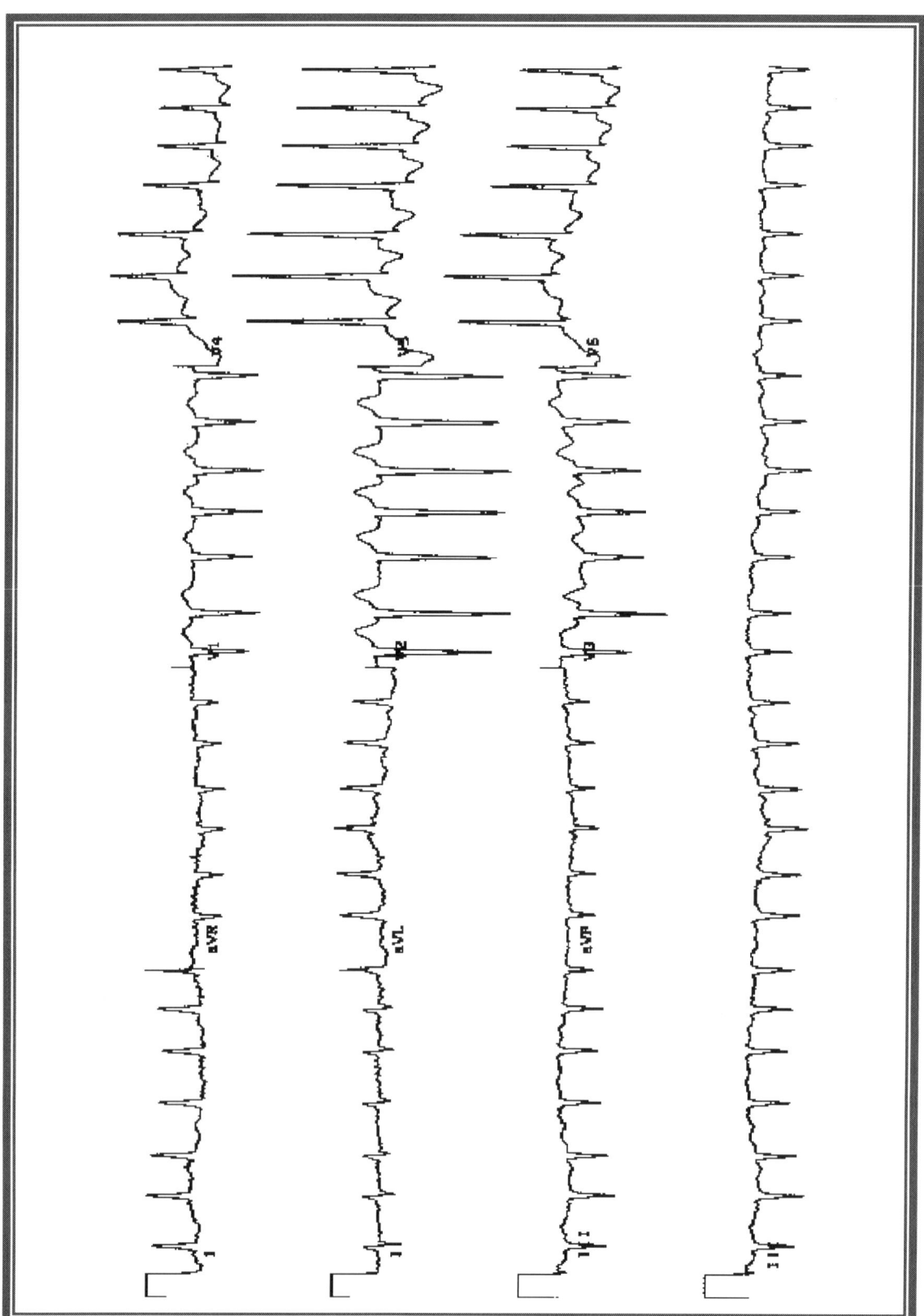

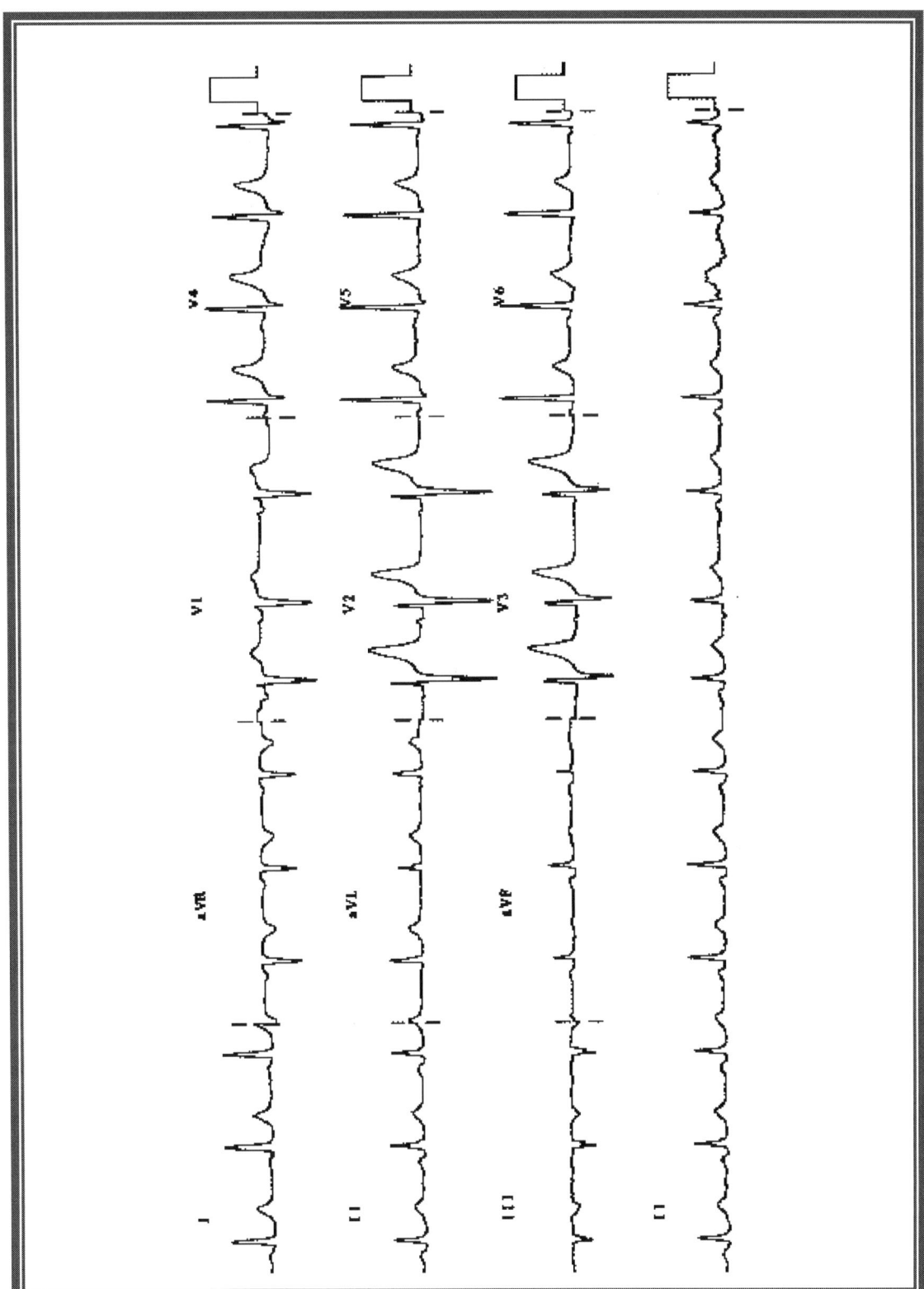

Write the Diagnosis of the previous EKG's:

1._____

2._____

3._____

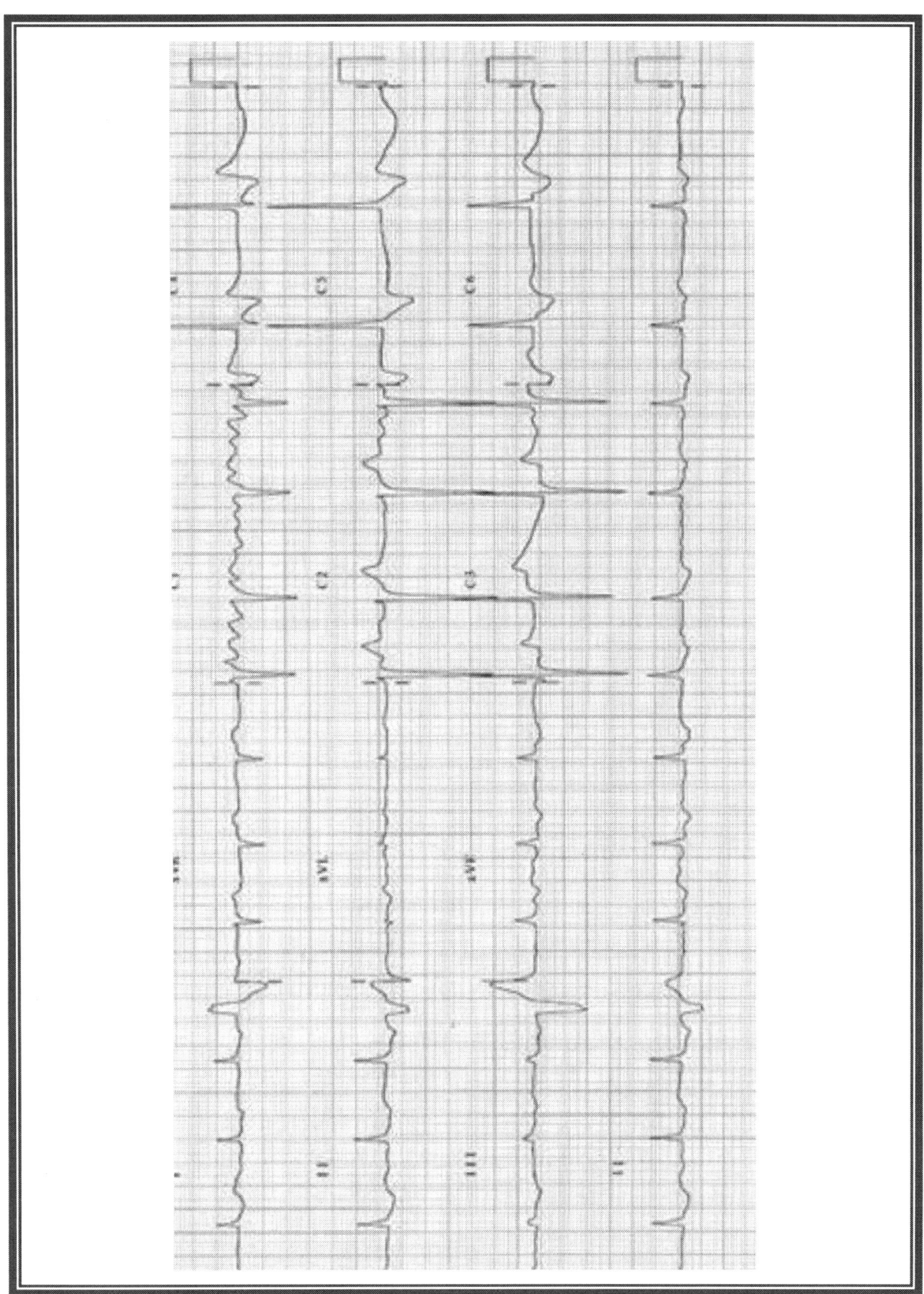

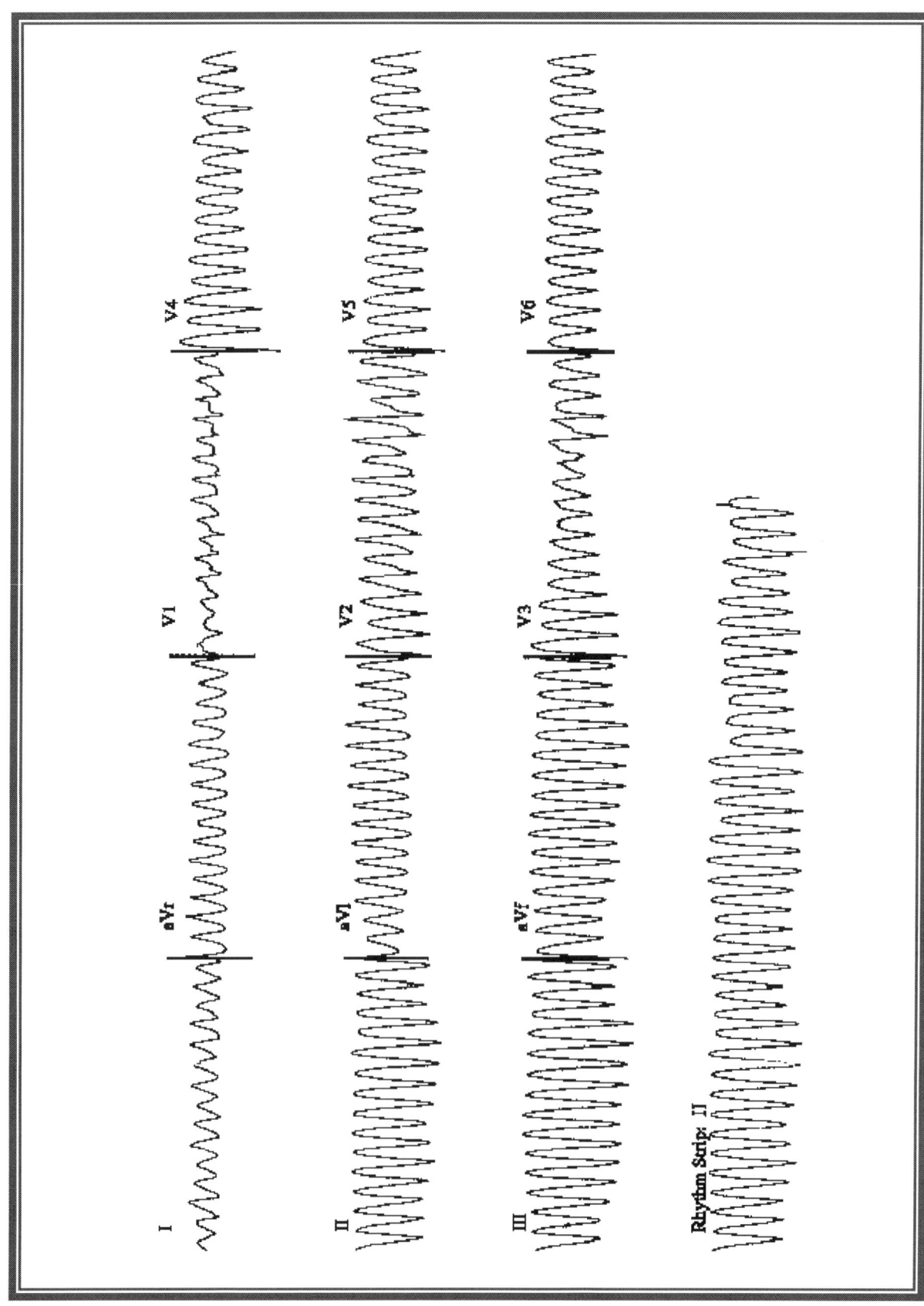

blank

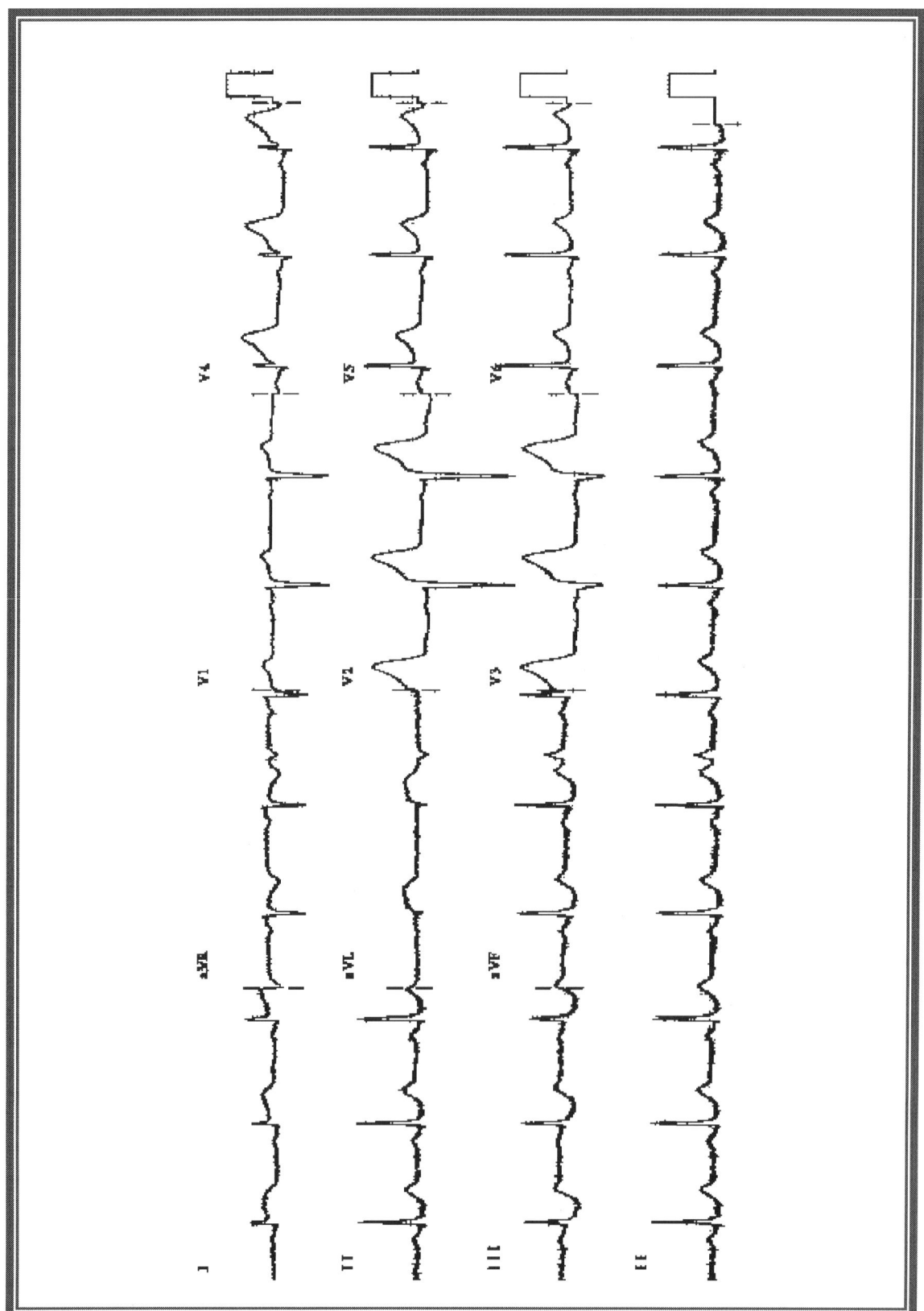

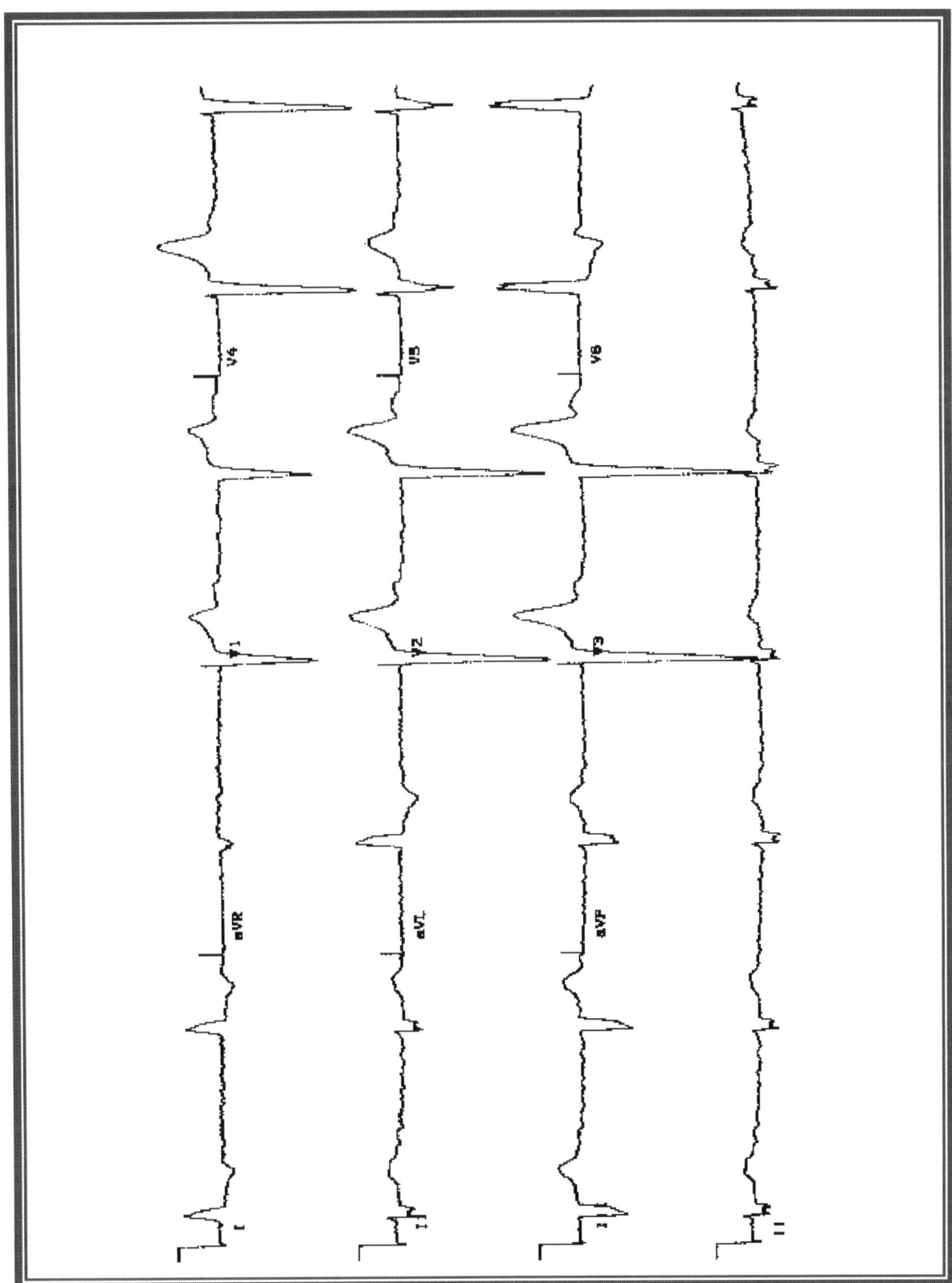

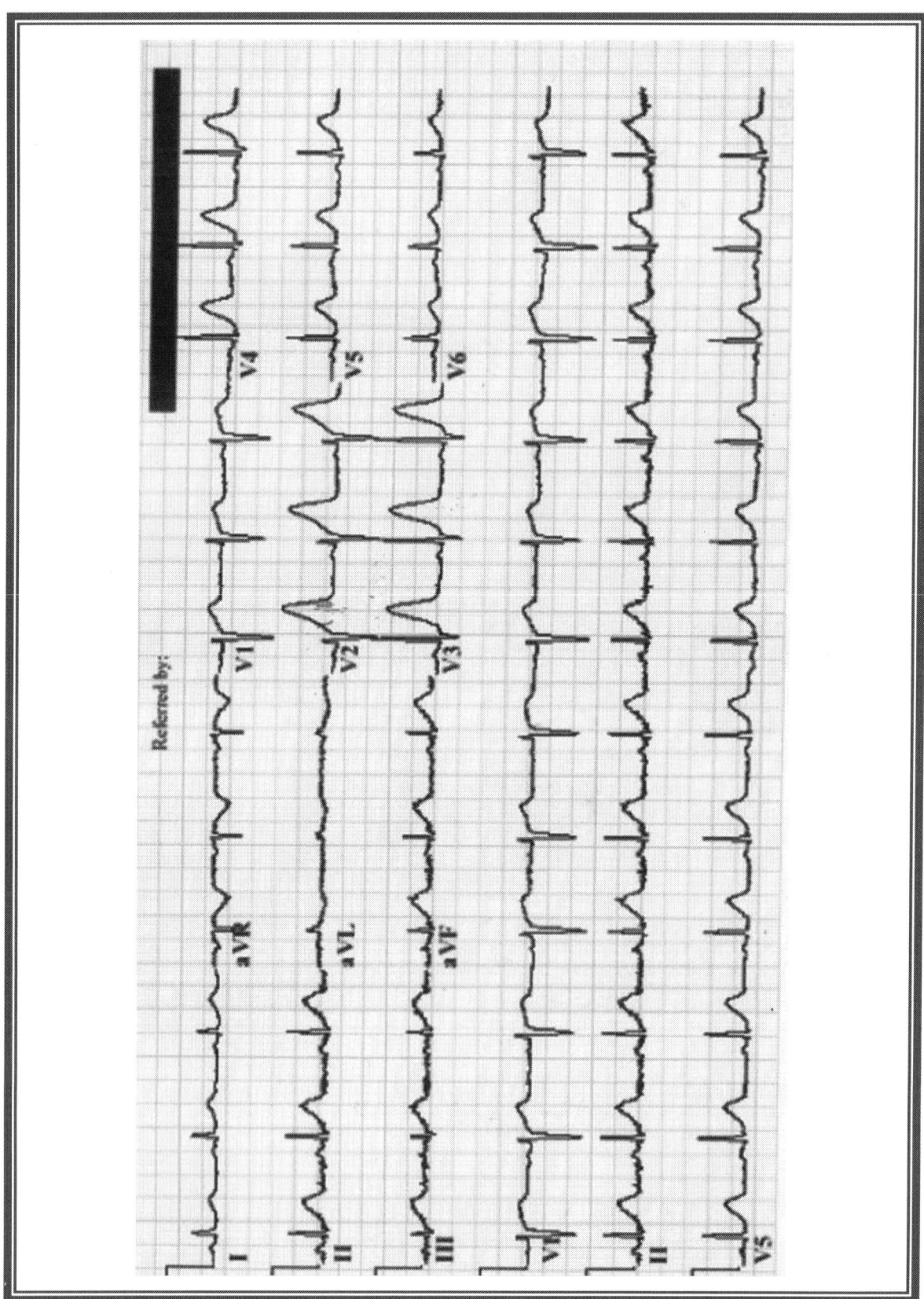

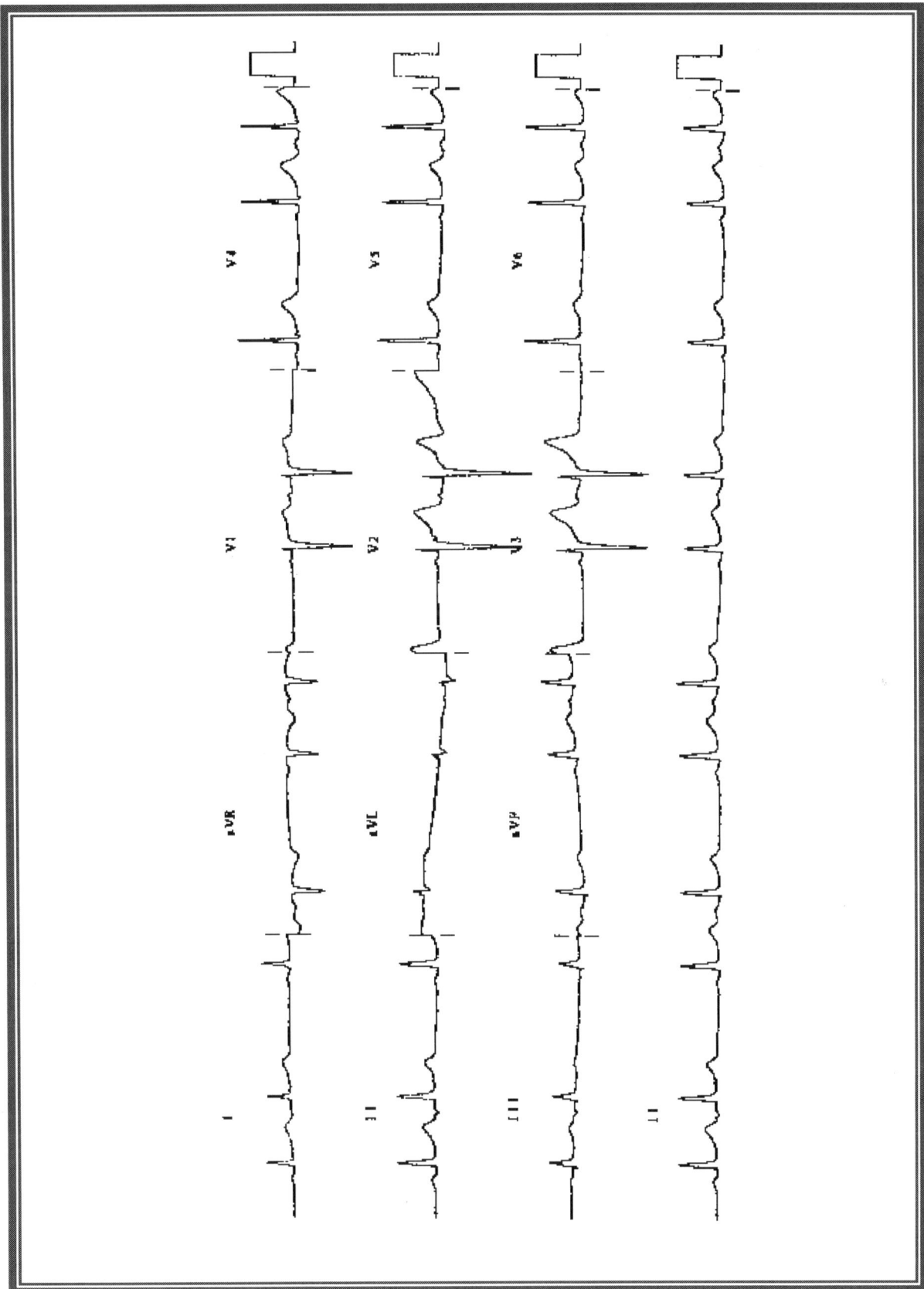

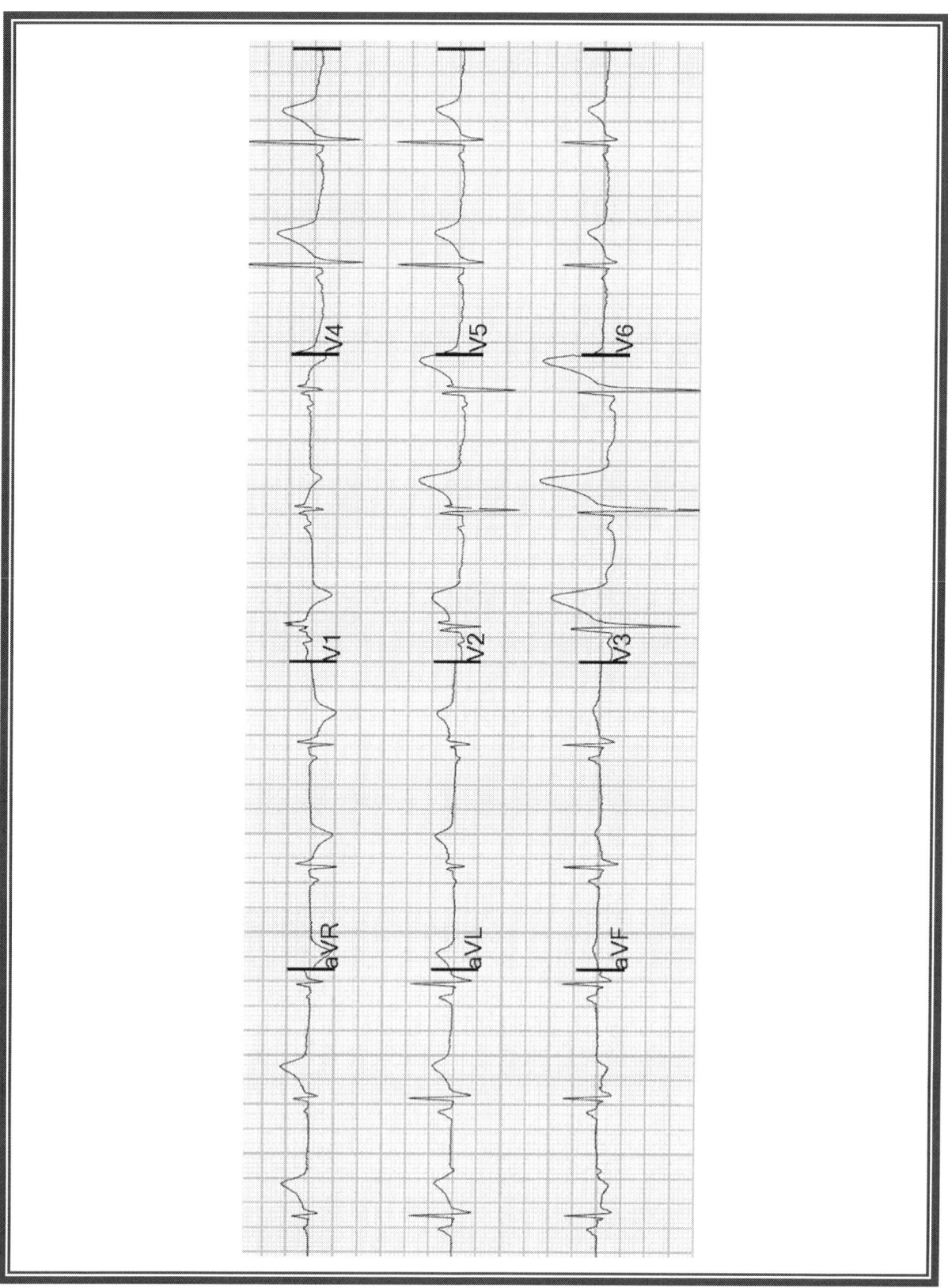

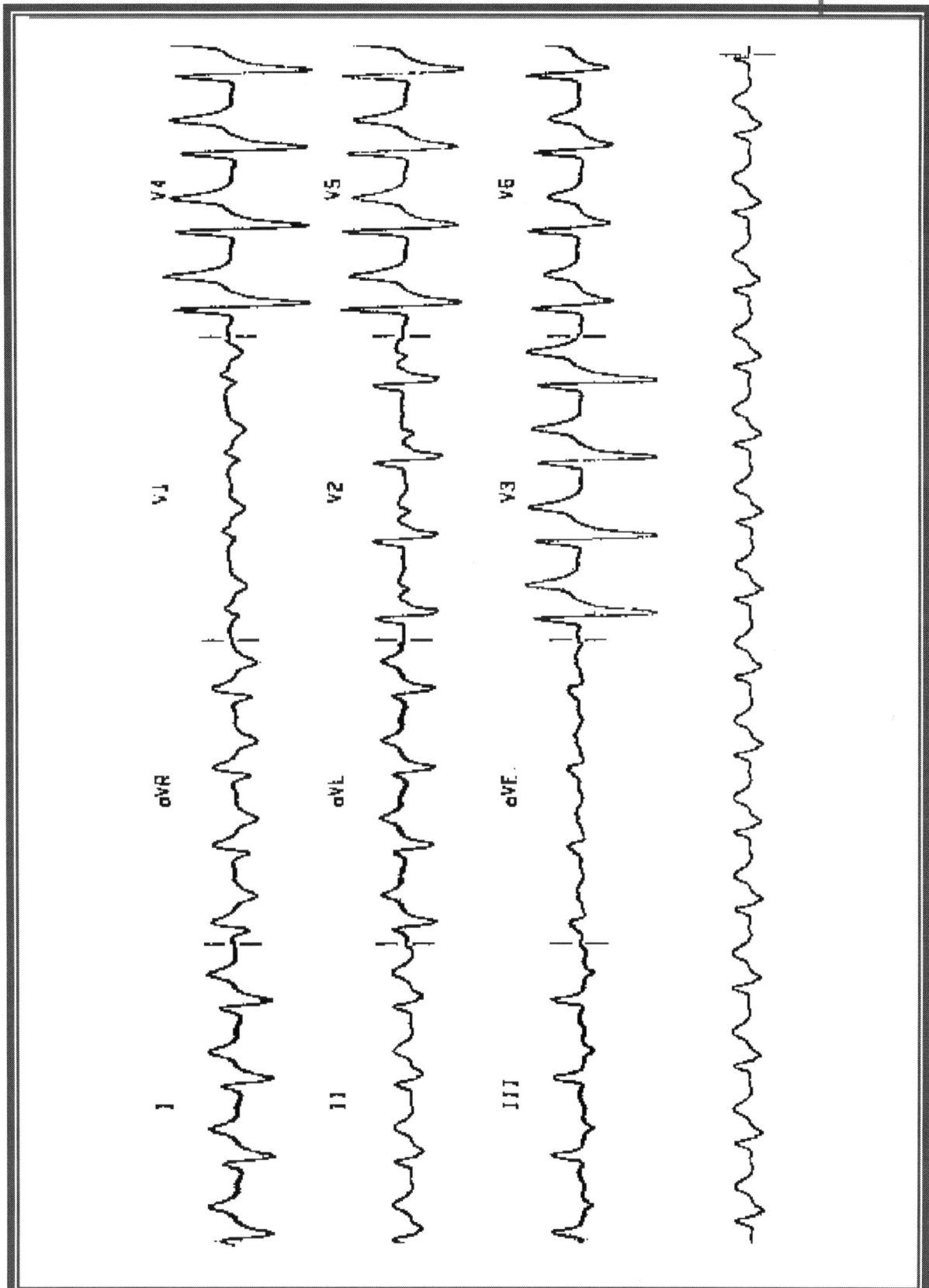

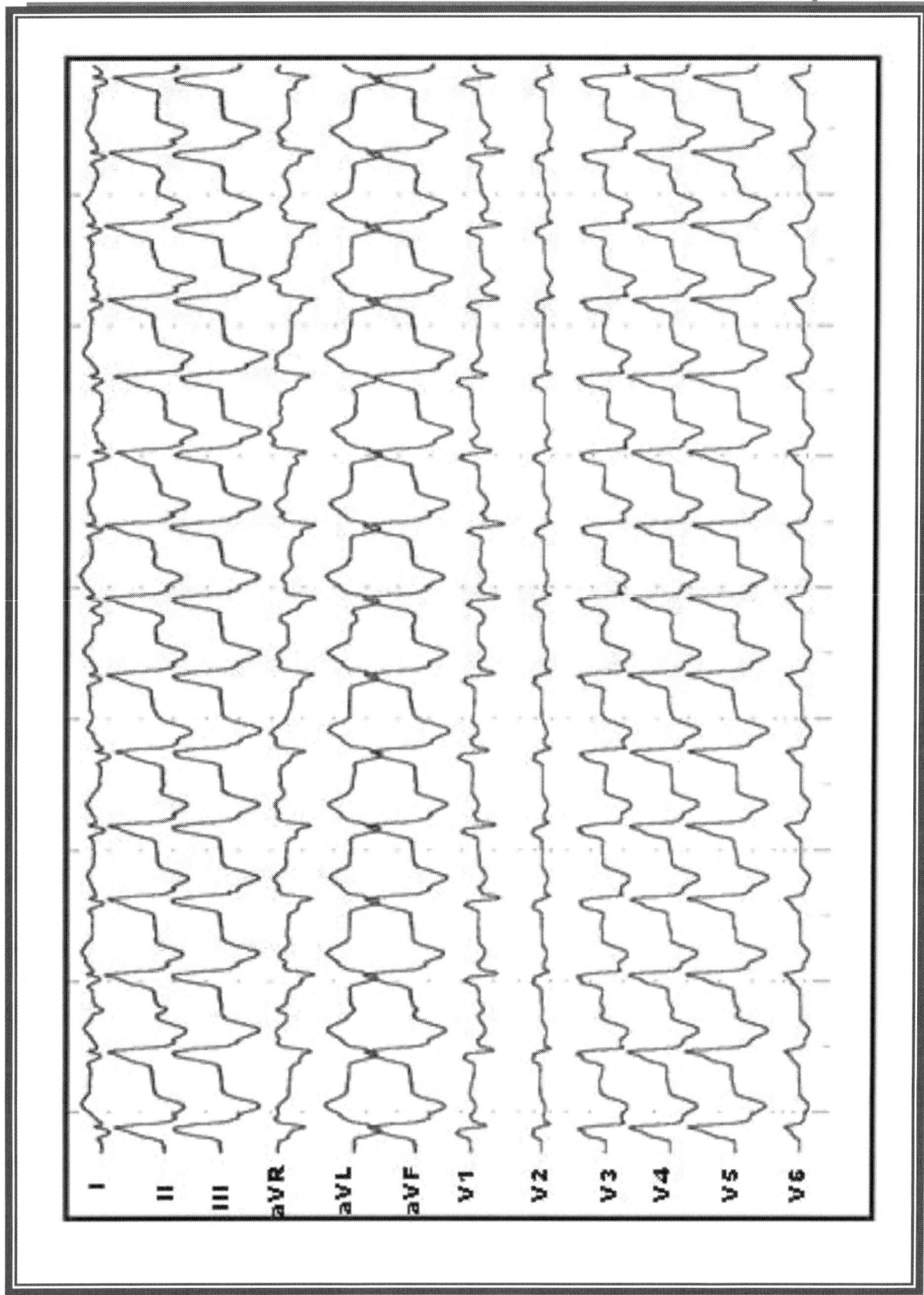

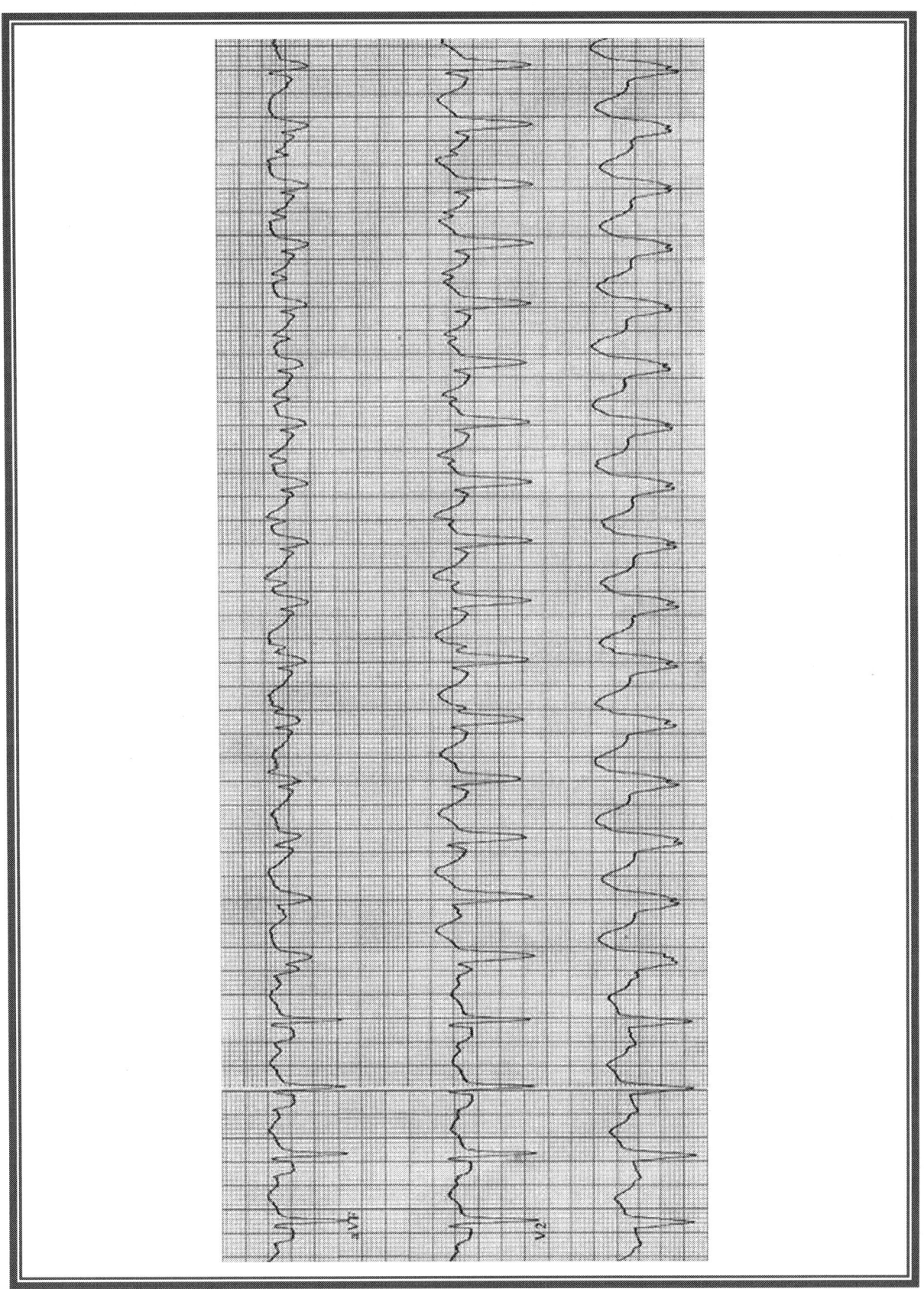

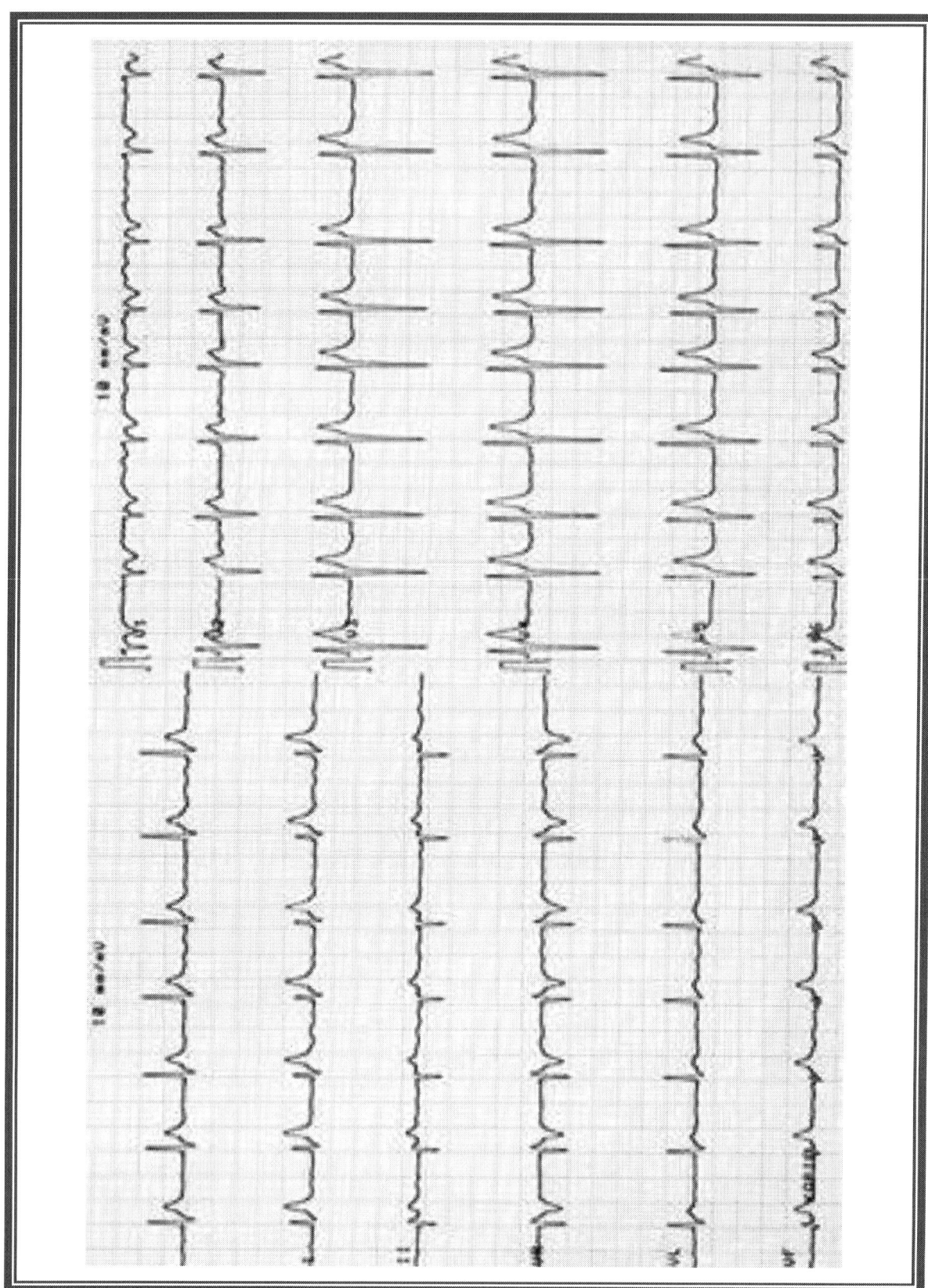

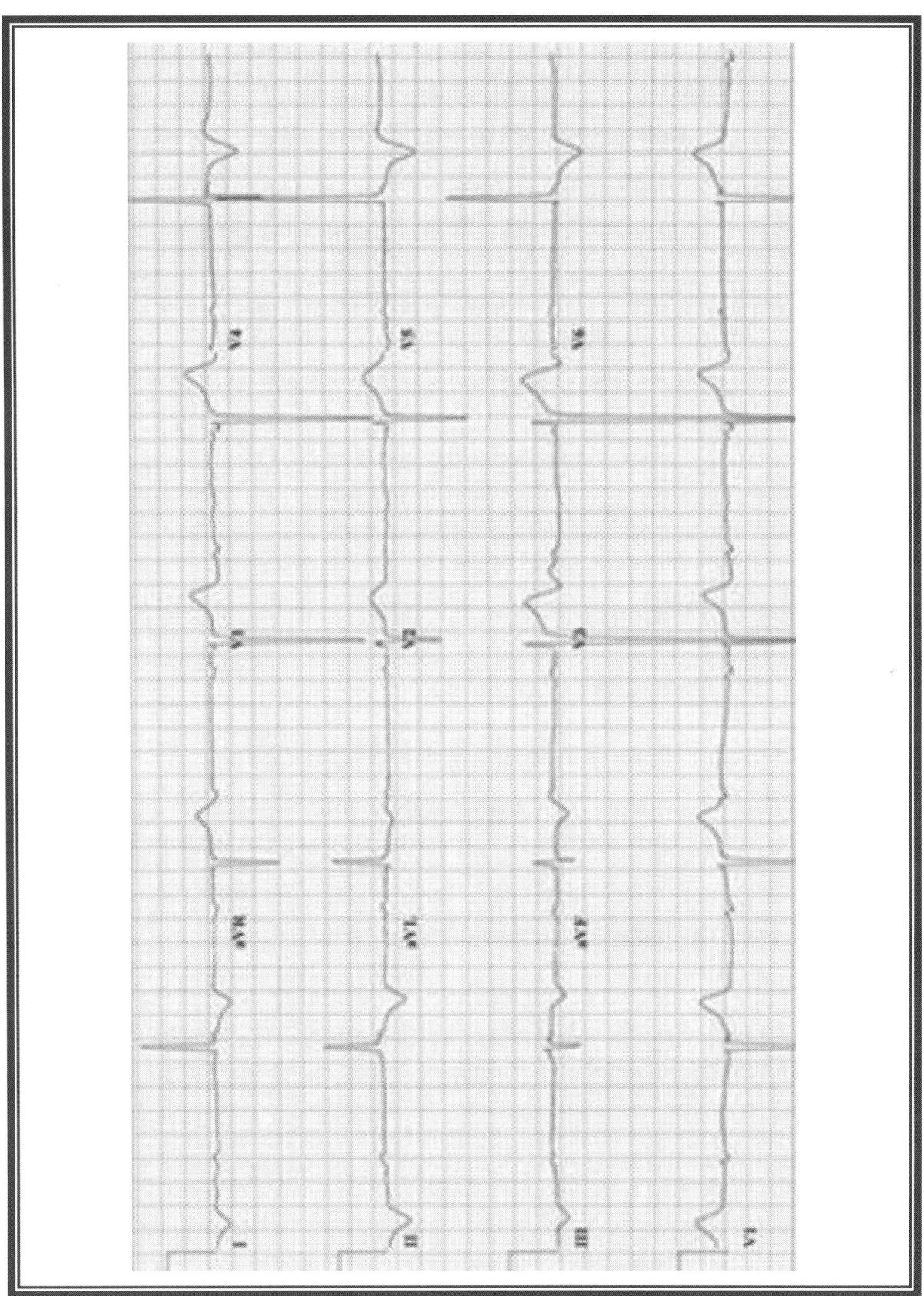

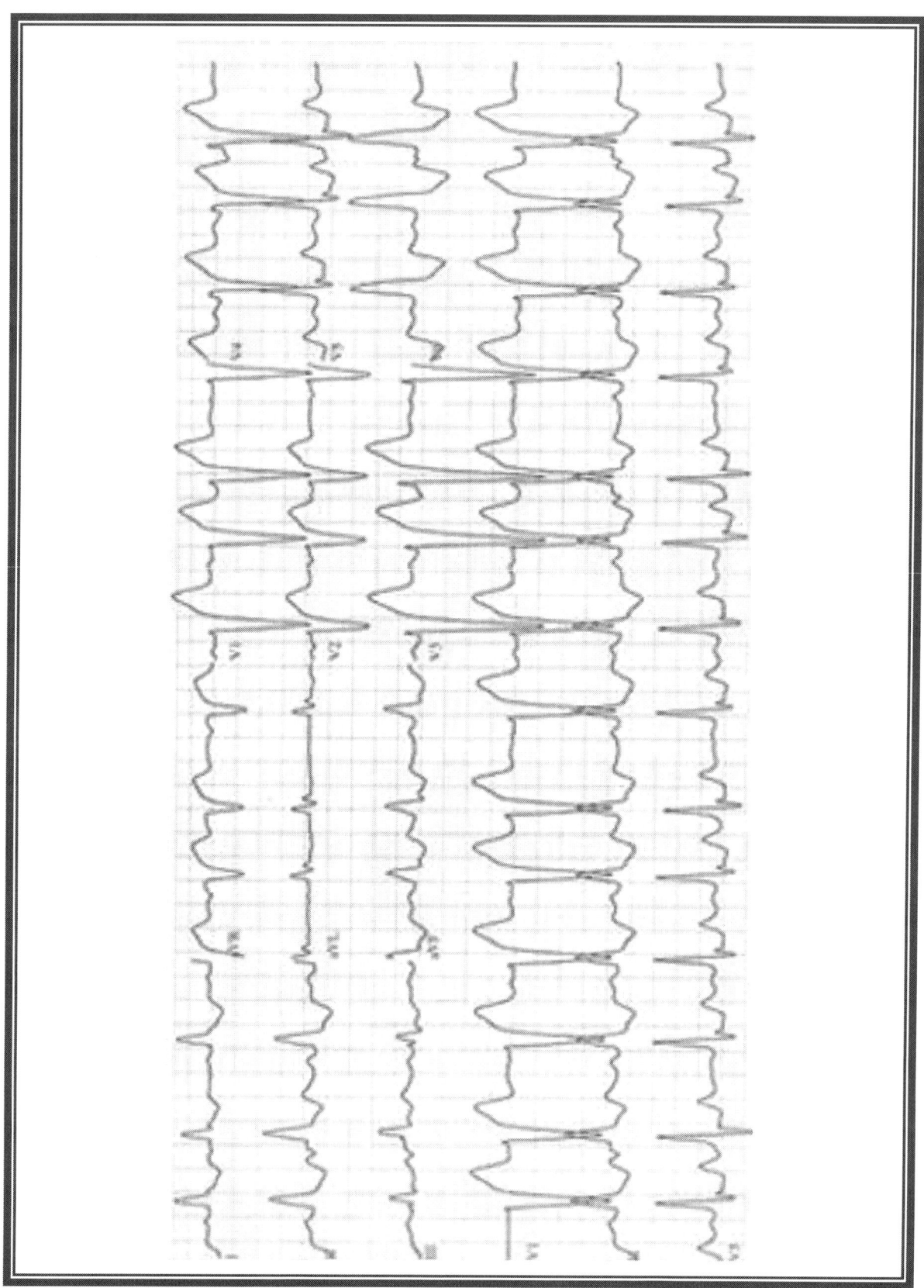

Write the Diagnosis of the previous EKG's:

1._____

2._____

3._____

4._____

5._____

6._____

7._____

8._____

9._____

10._____

11._____

12._____

13._____

14._____

15._____

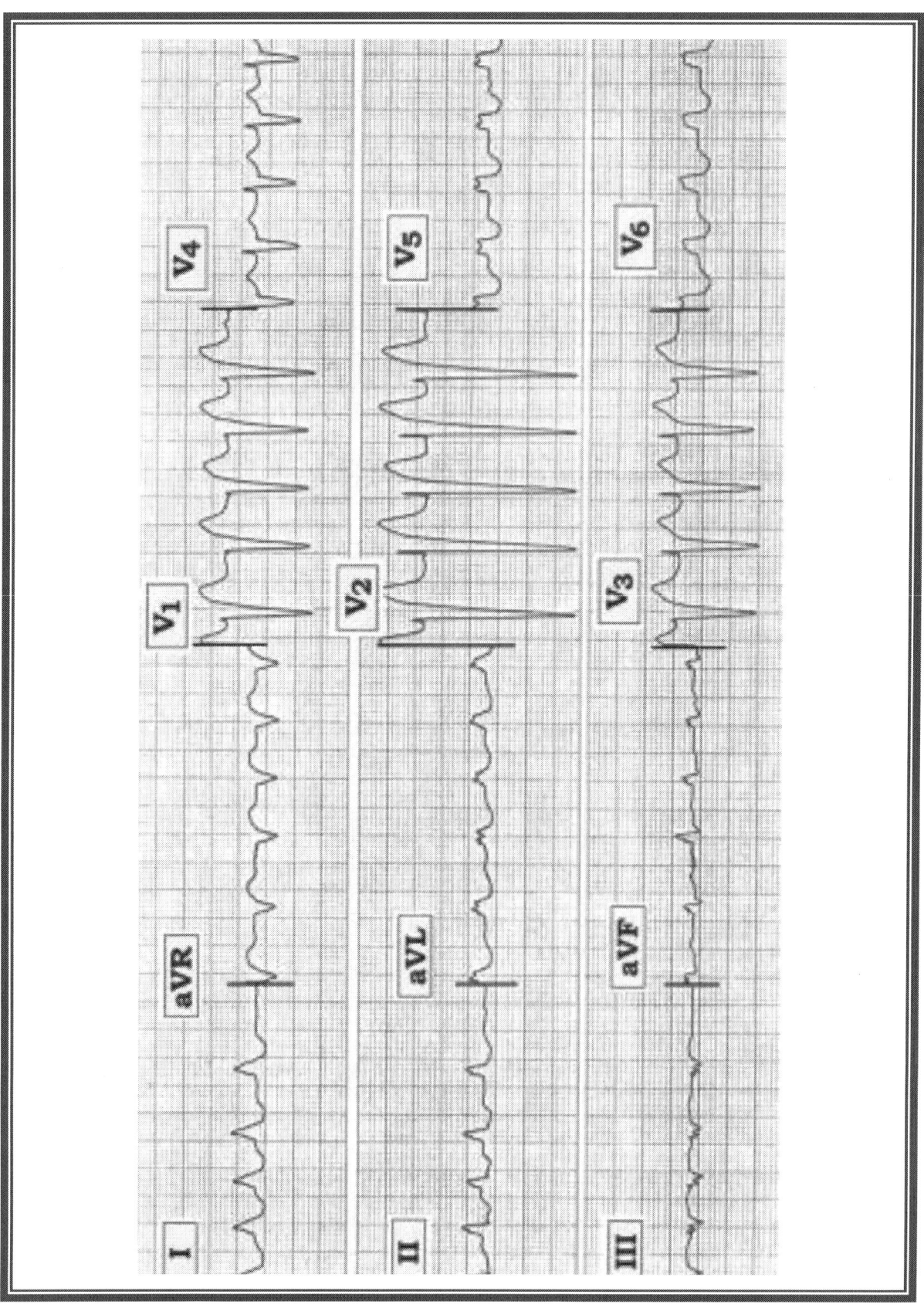

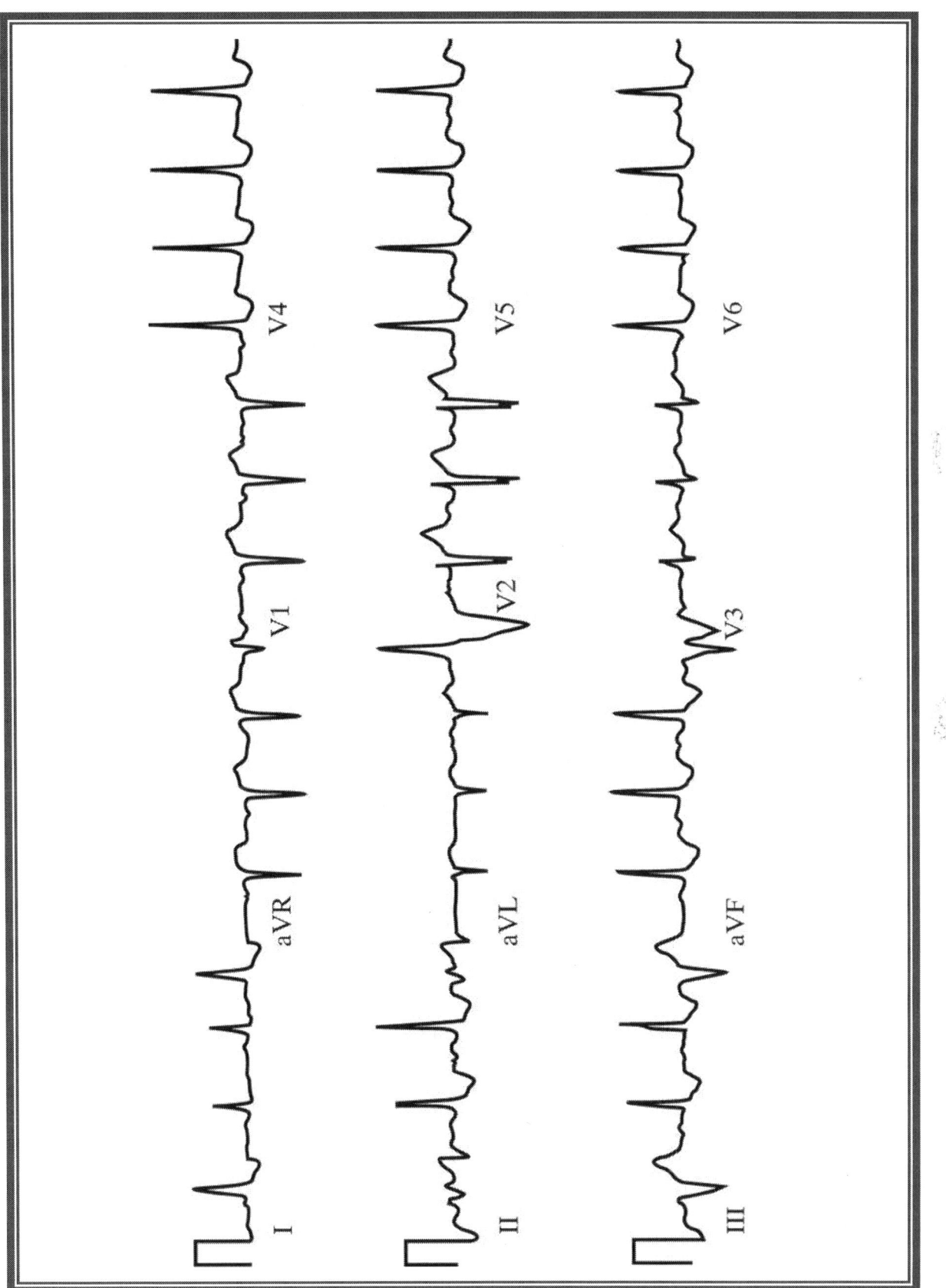

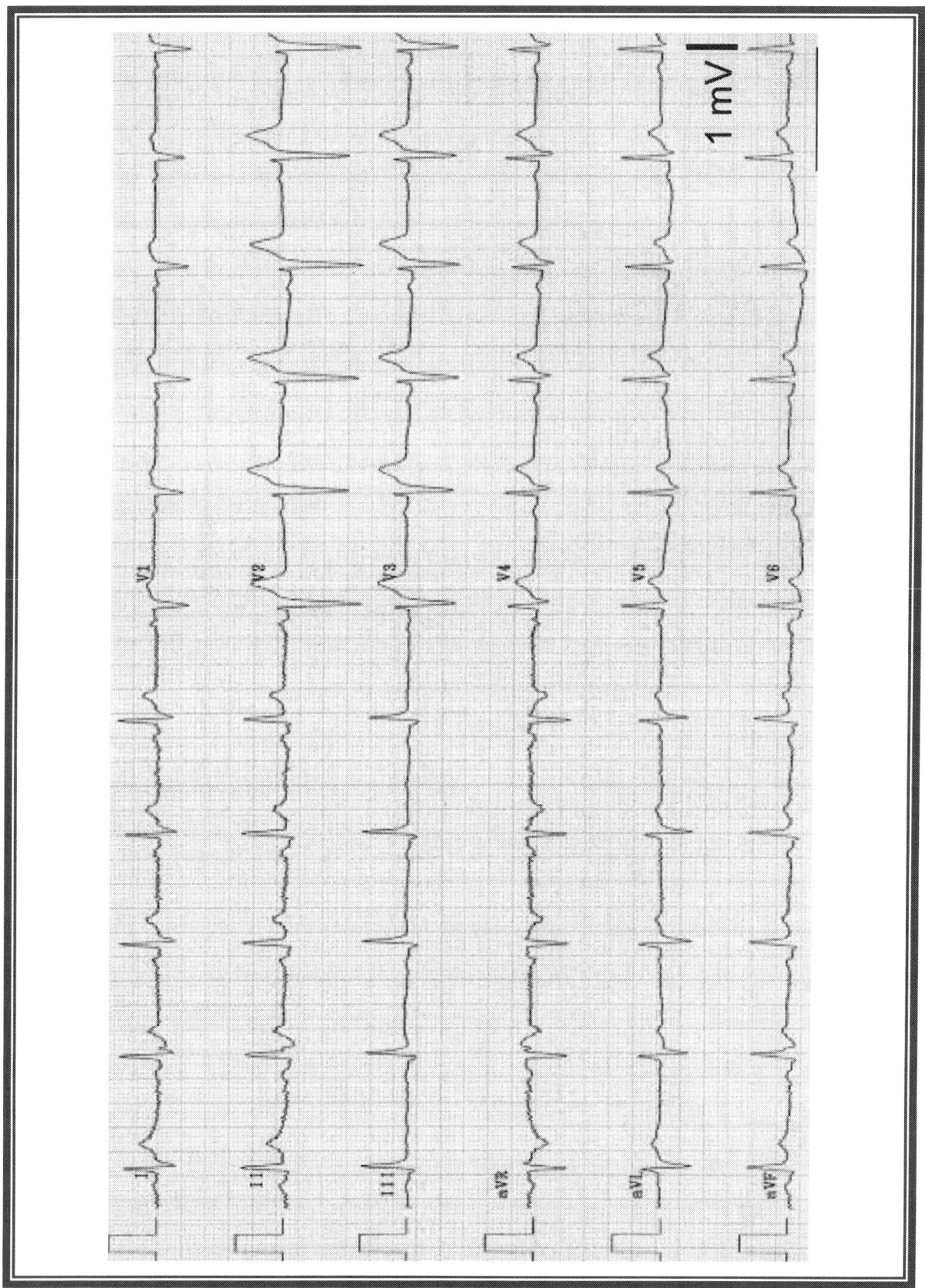

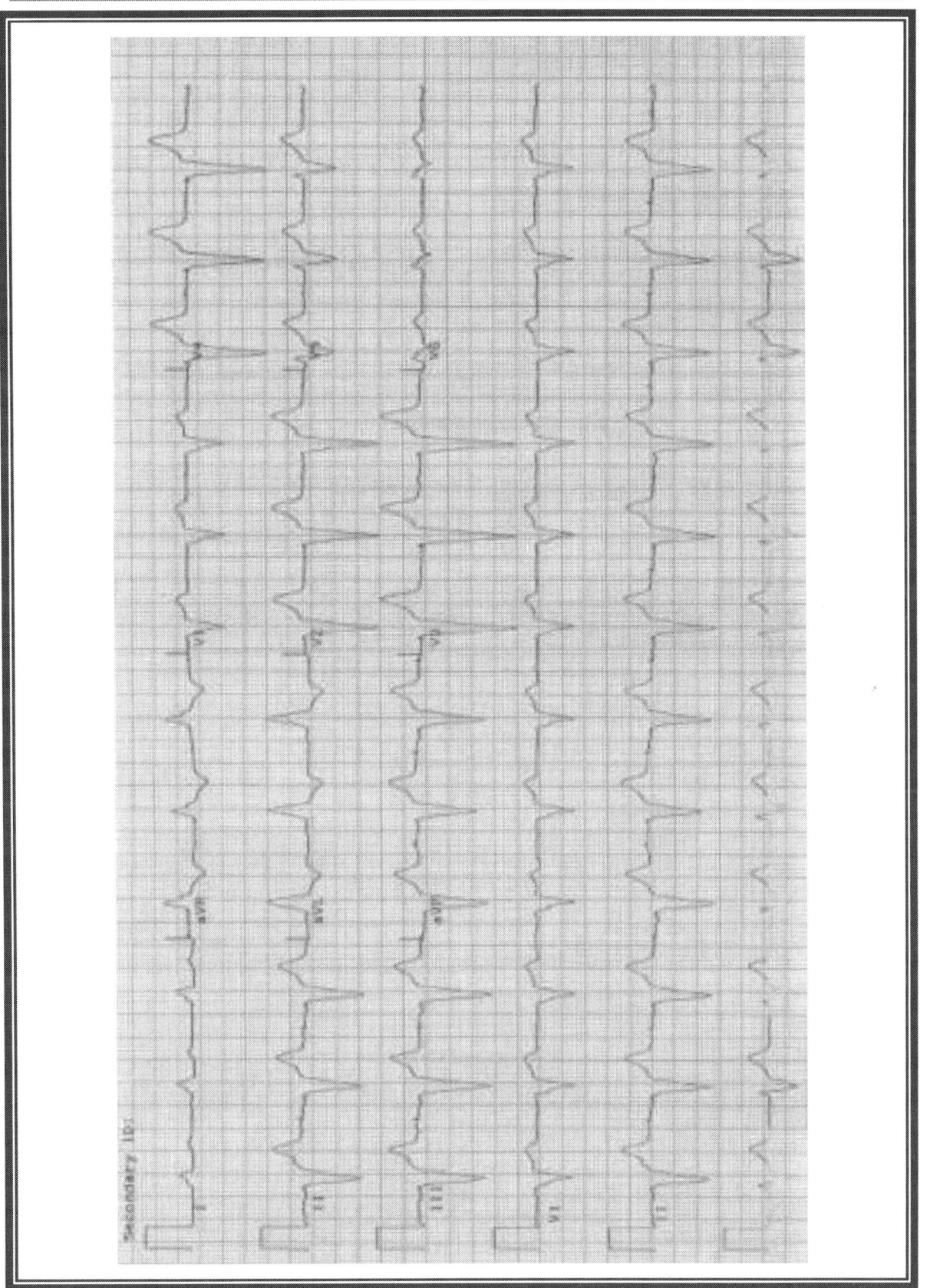

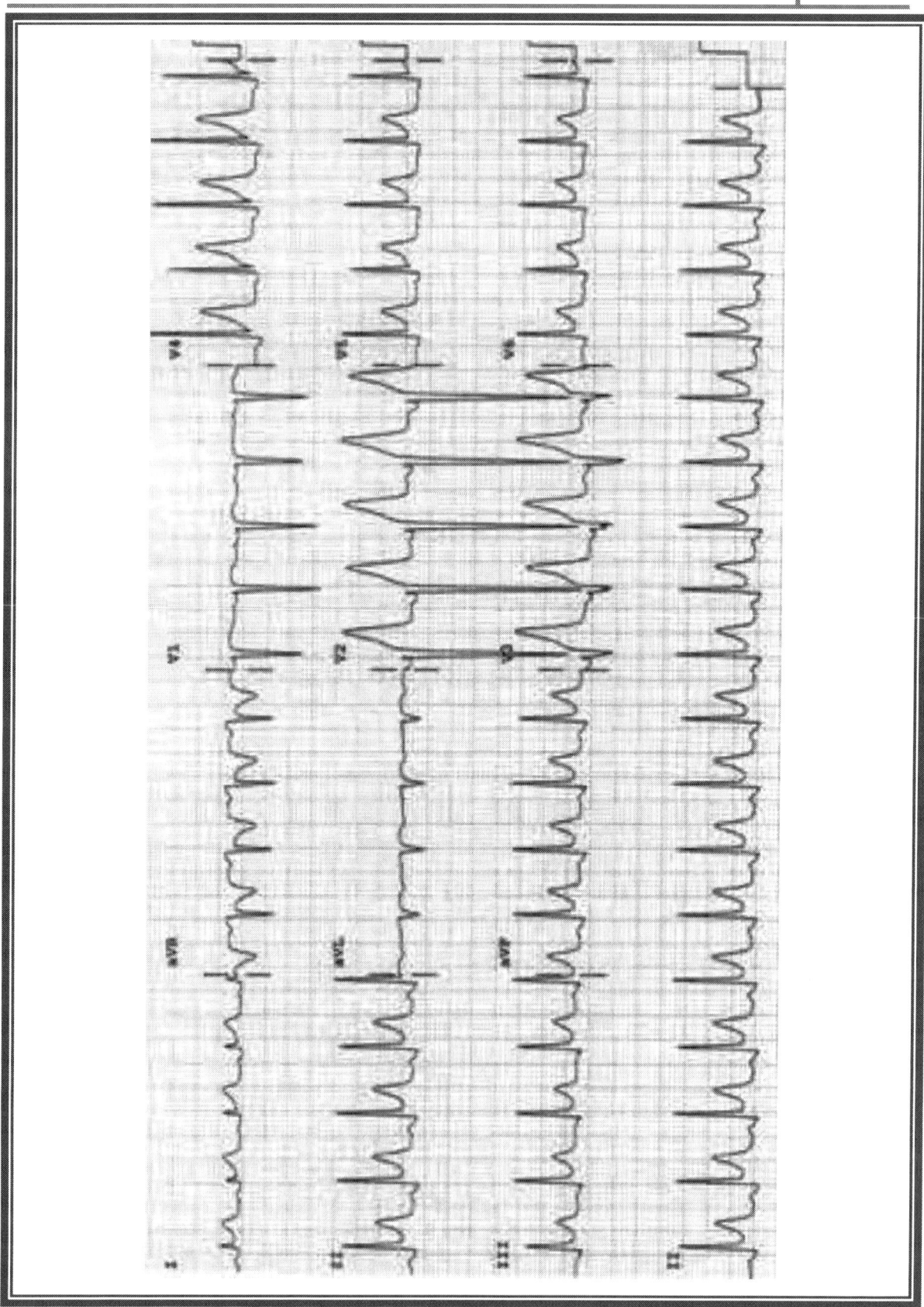

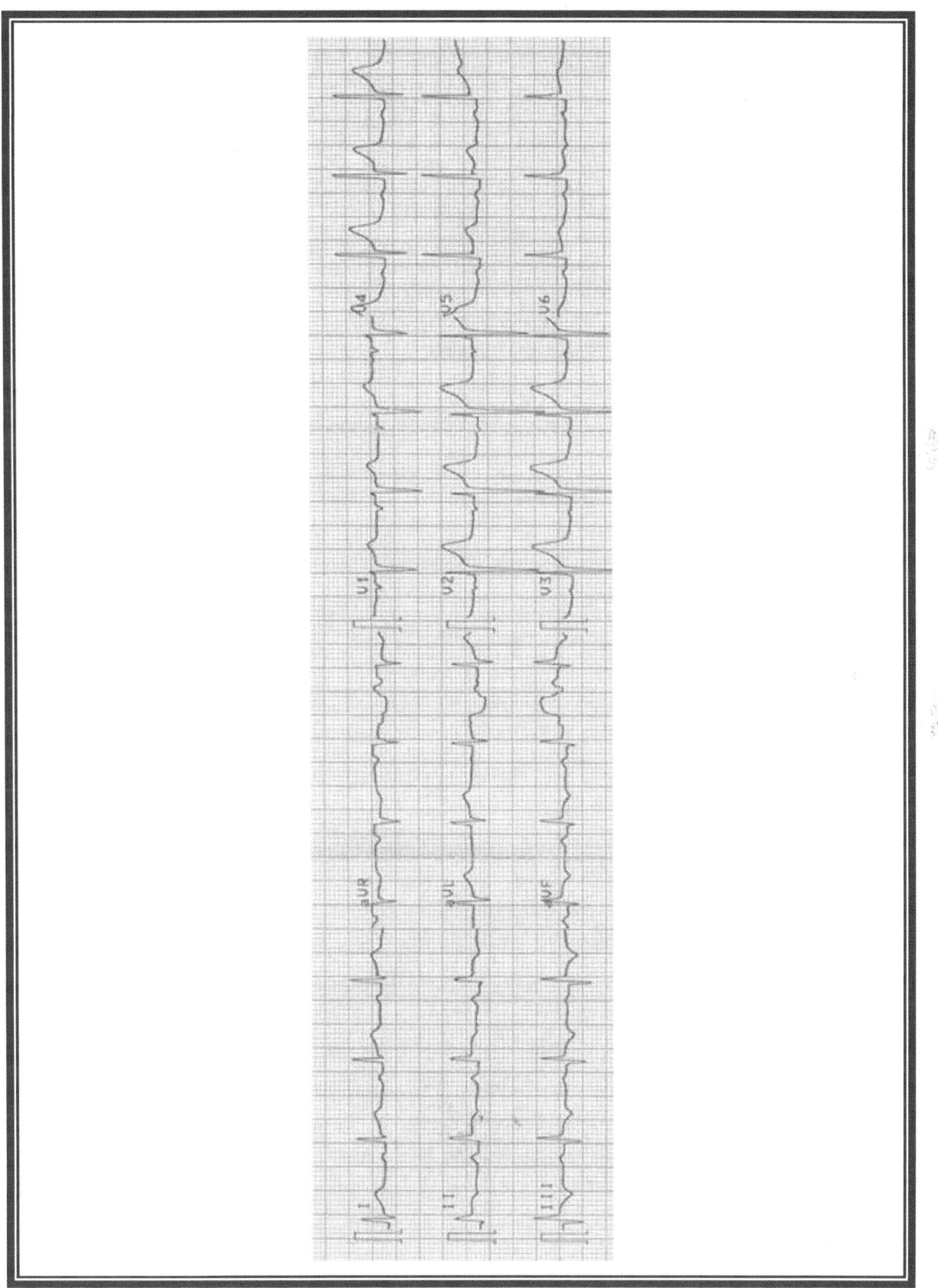

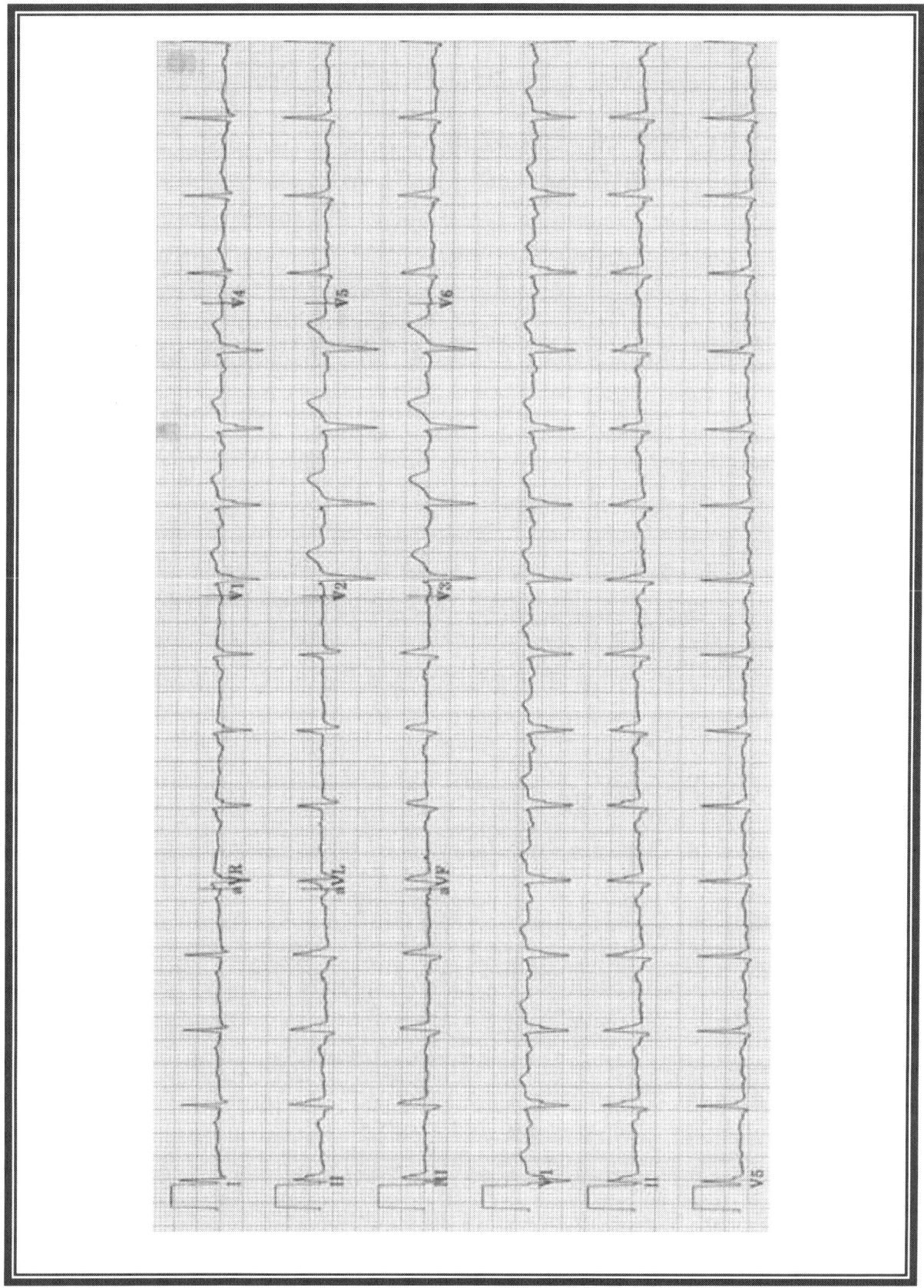

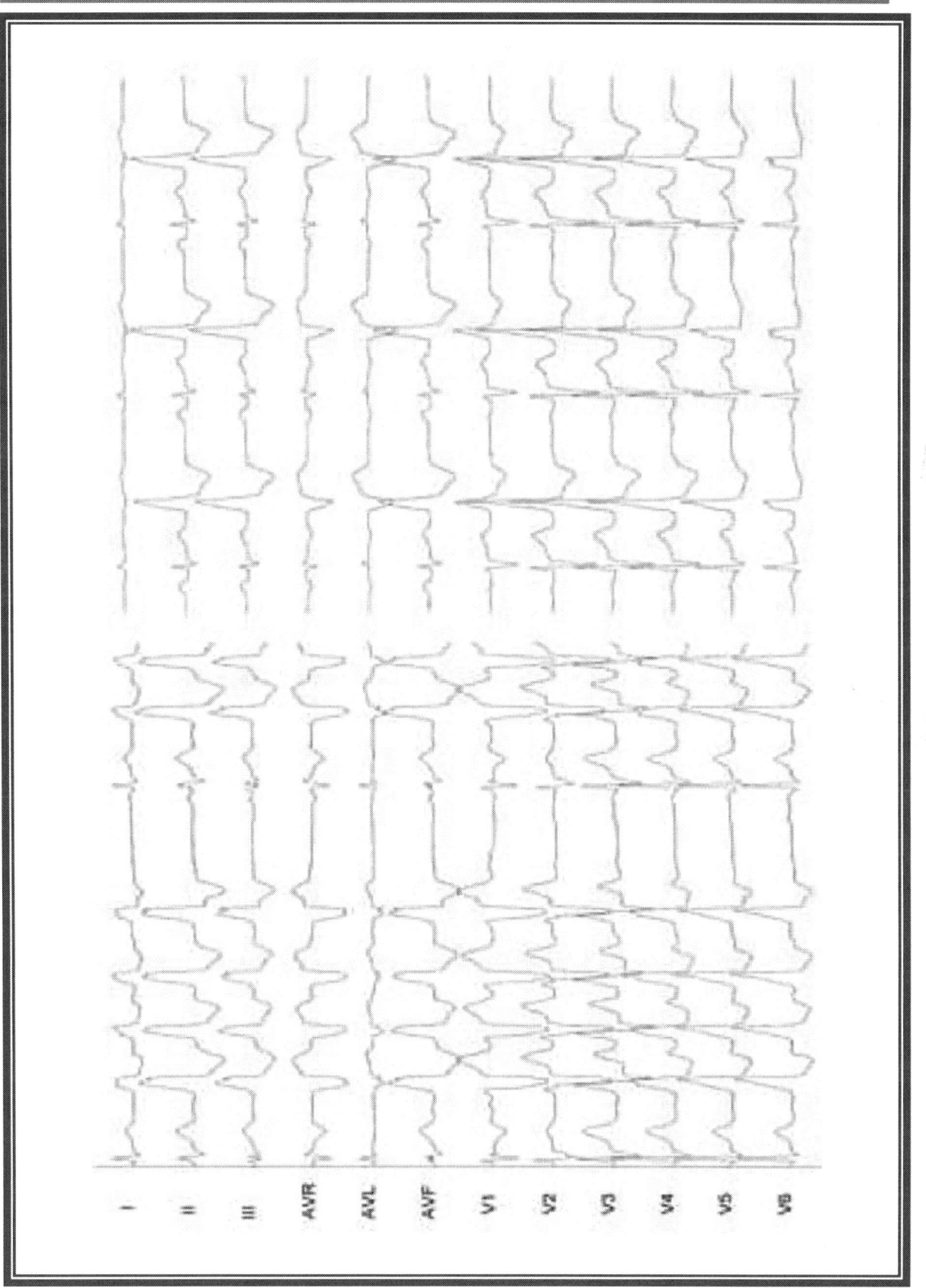

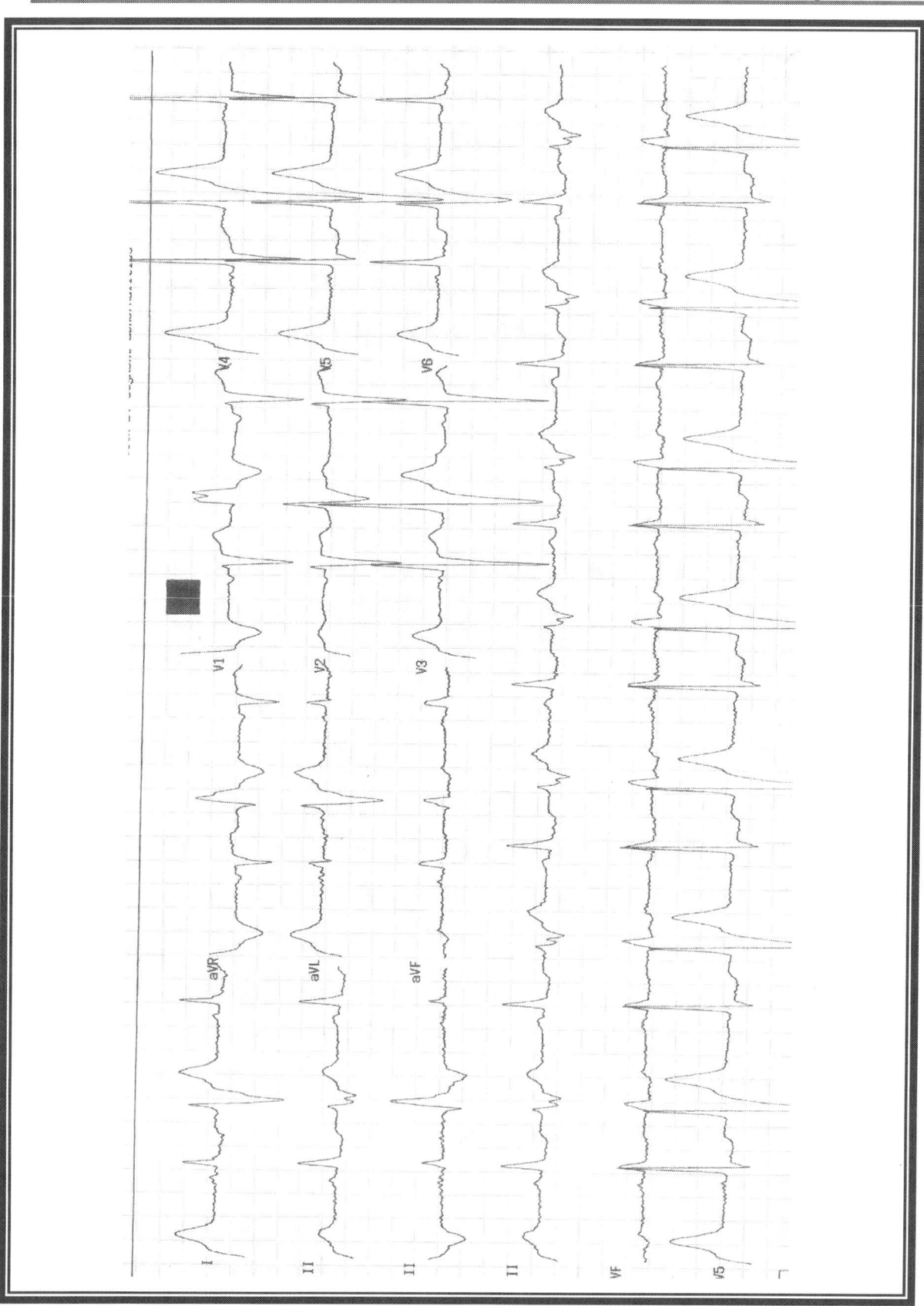

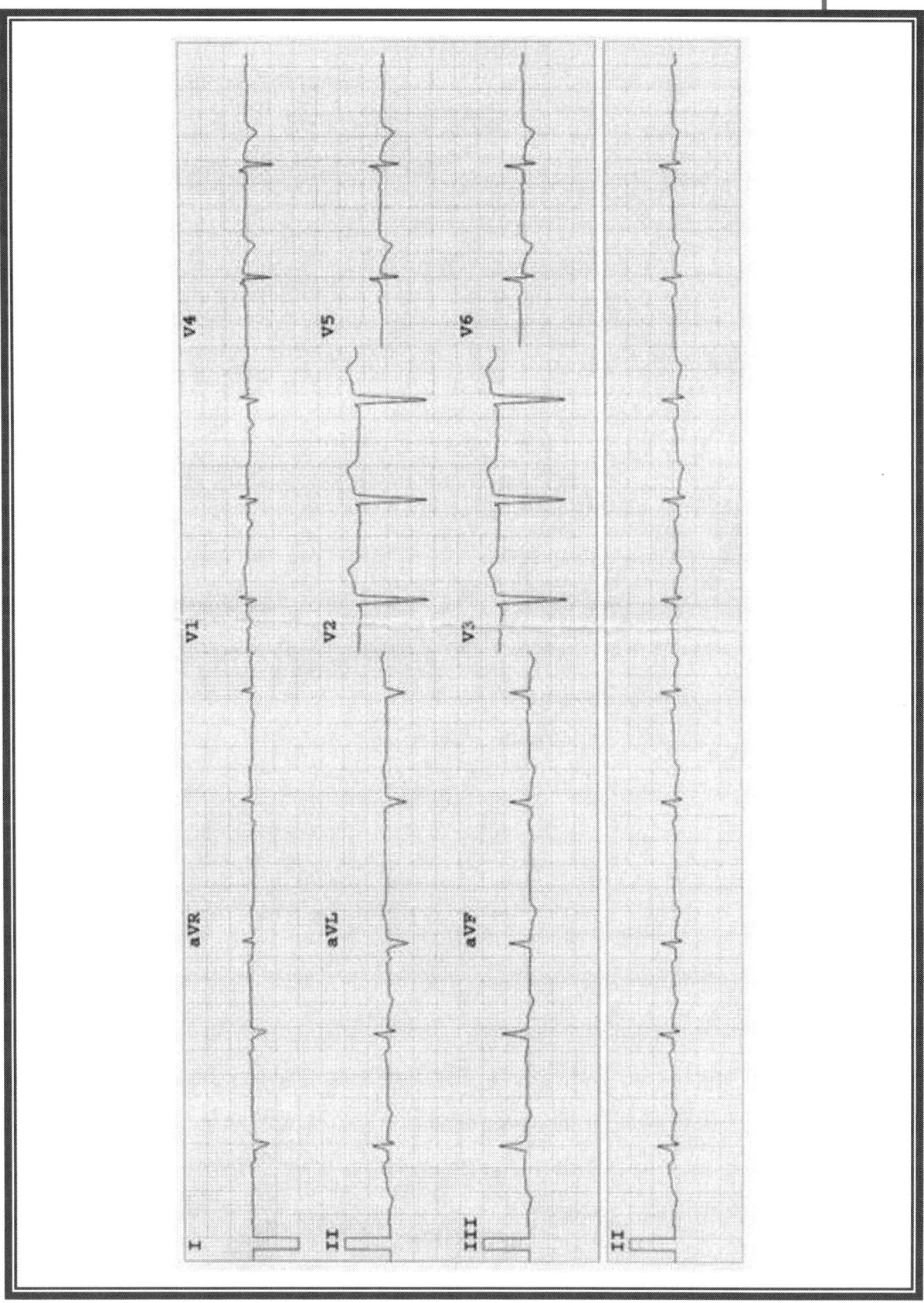

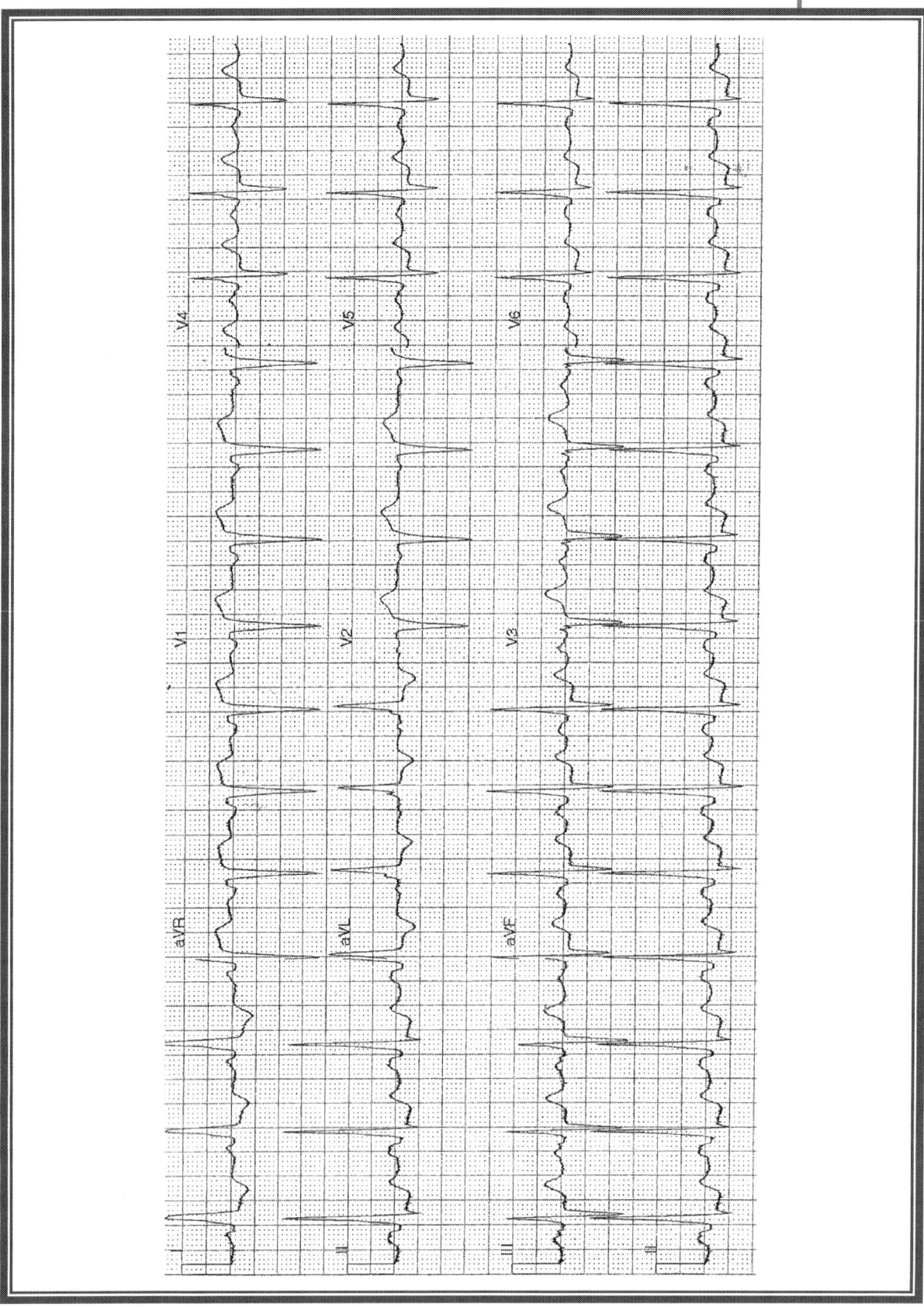

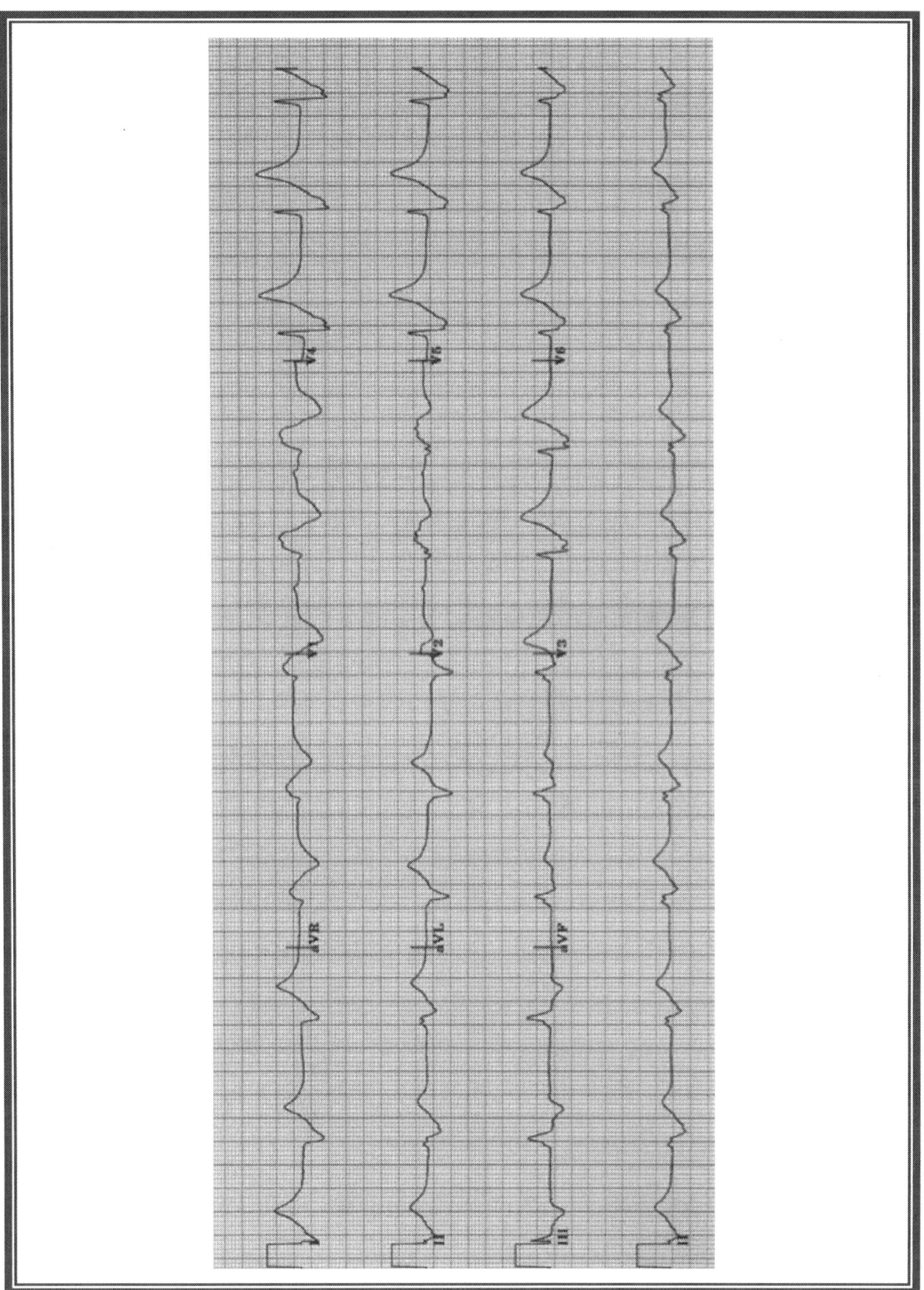

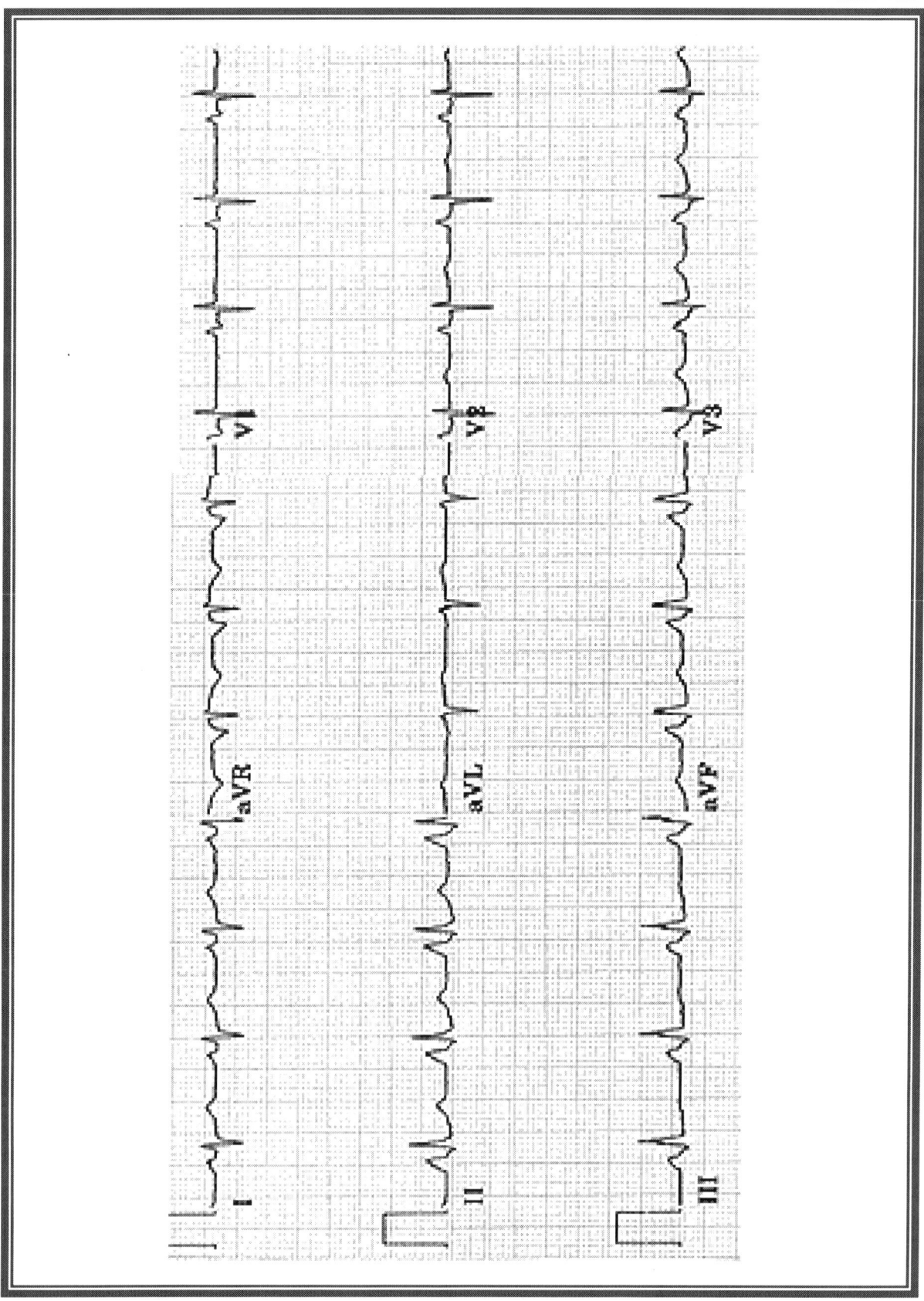

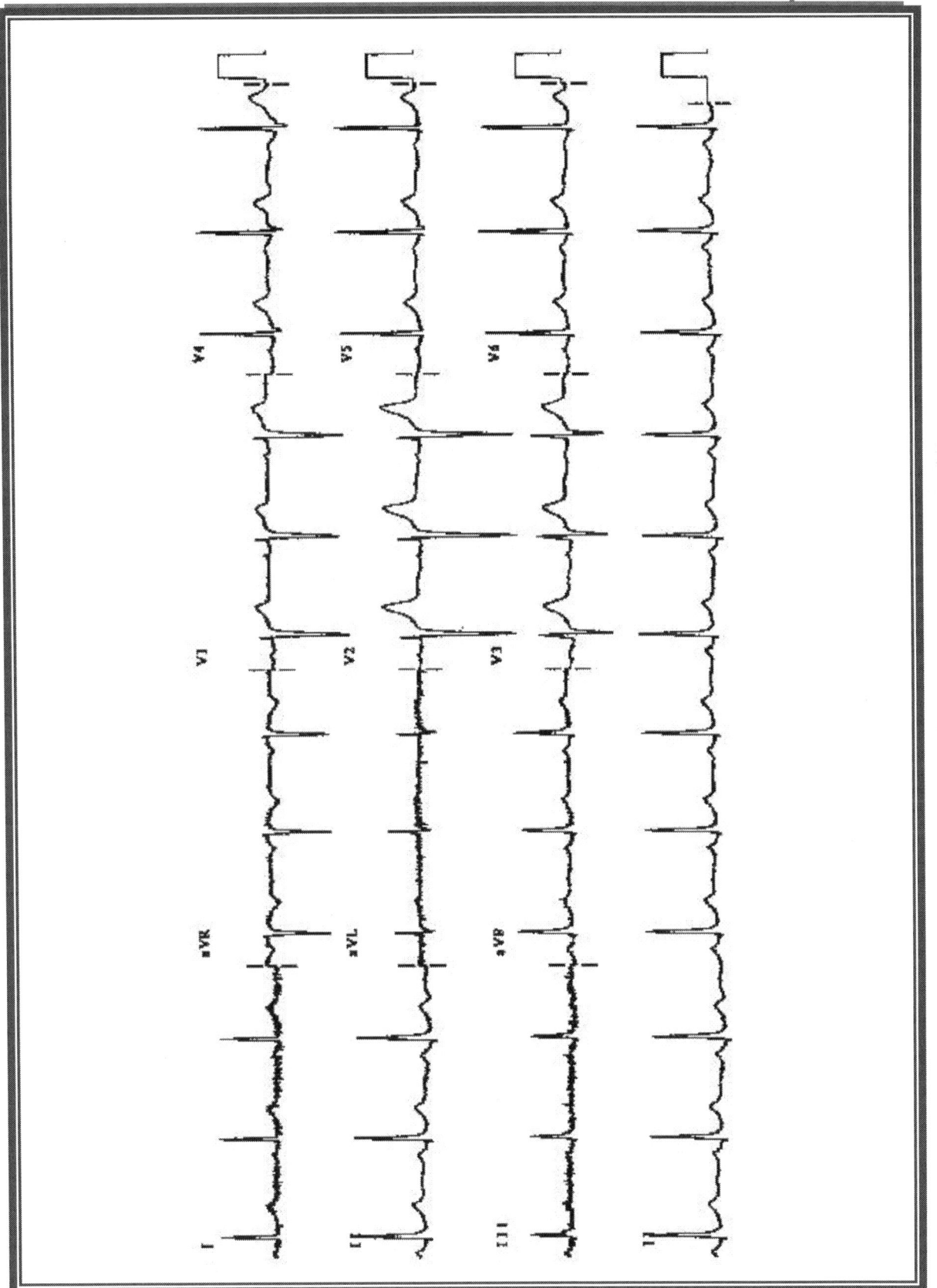

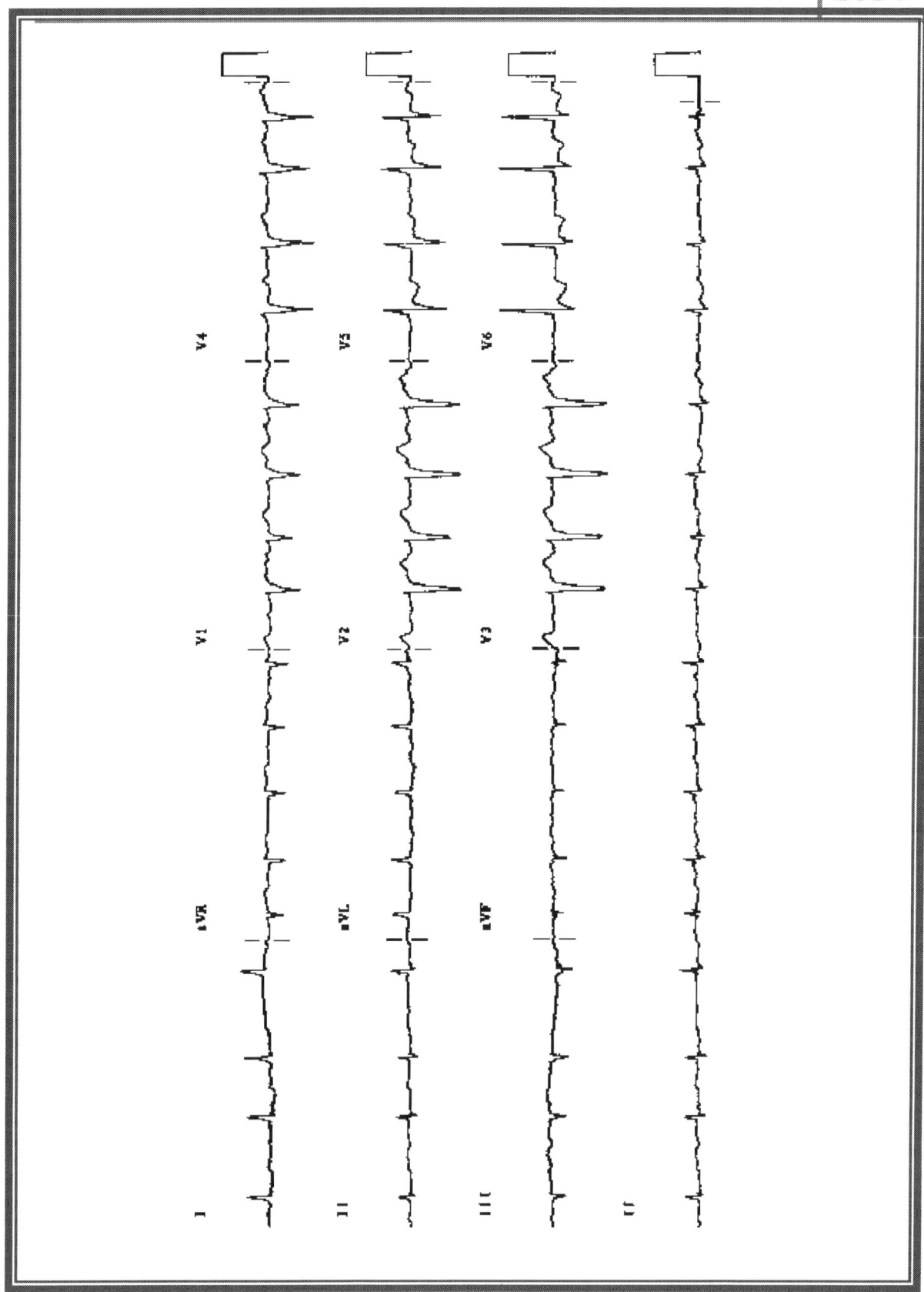

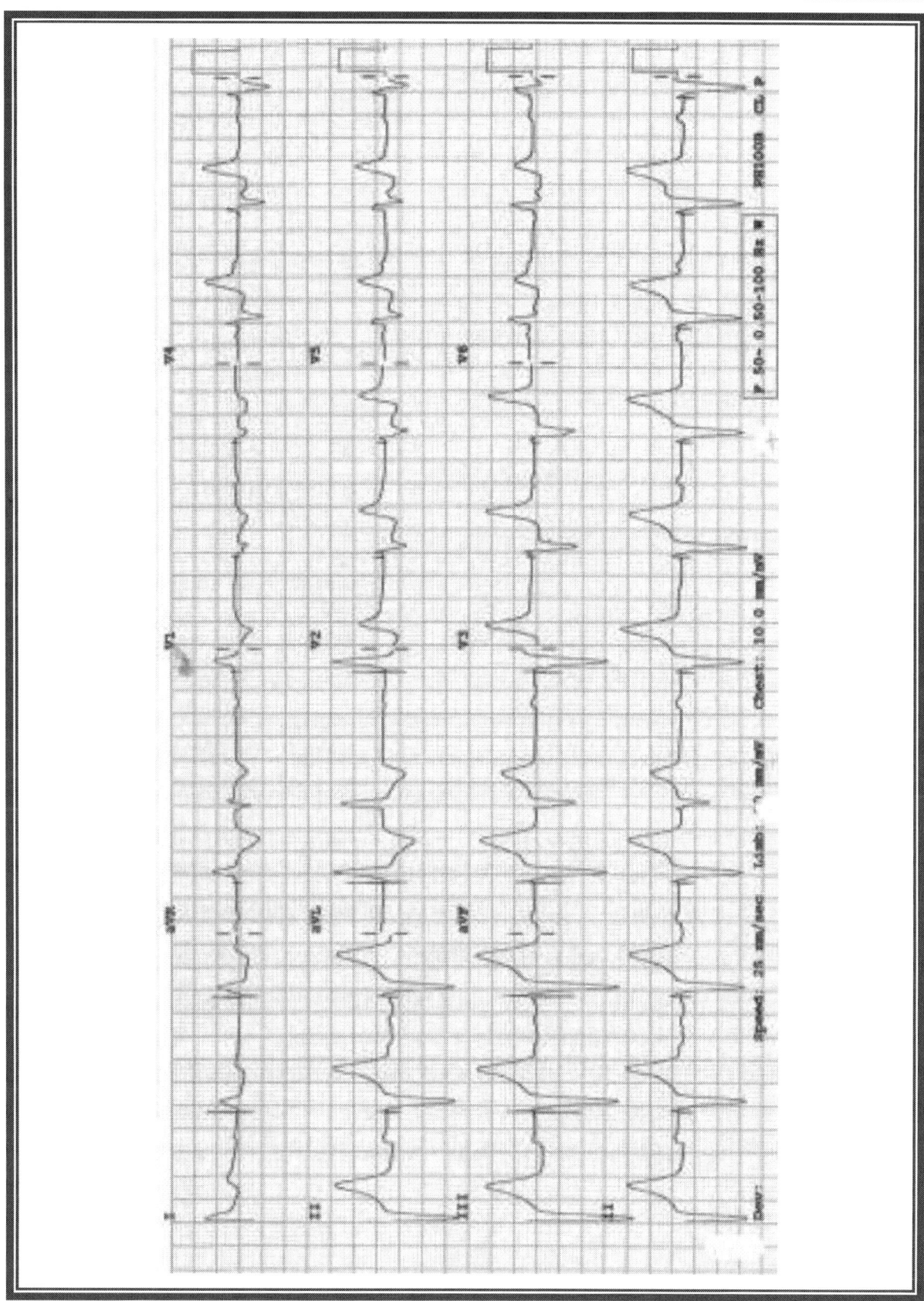

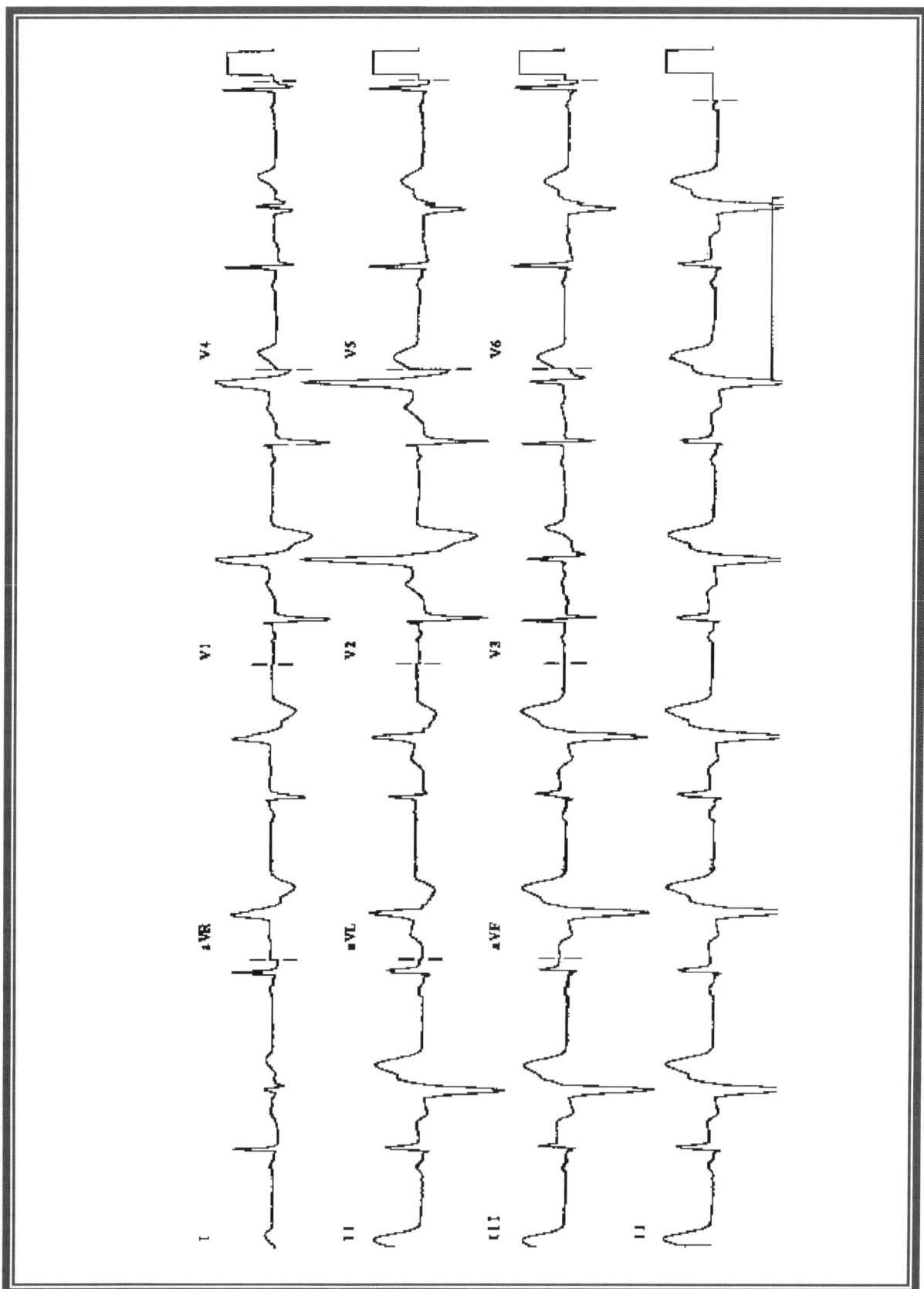

Write the Diagnosis of the previous EKG's:

1._____

2._____

3._____

4._____

5._____

6._____

7._____

8._____

9._____

10._____

11._____

12._____

13._____

14._____

15._____

16._____

17._____

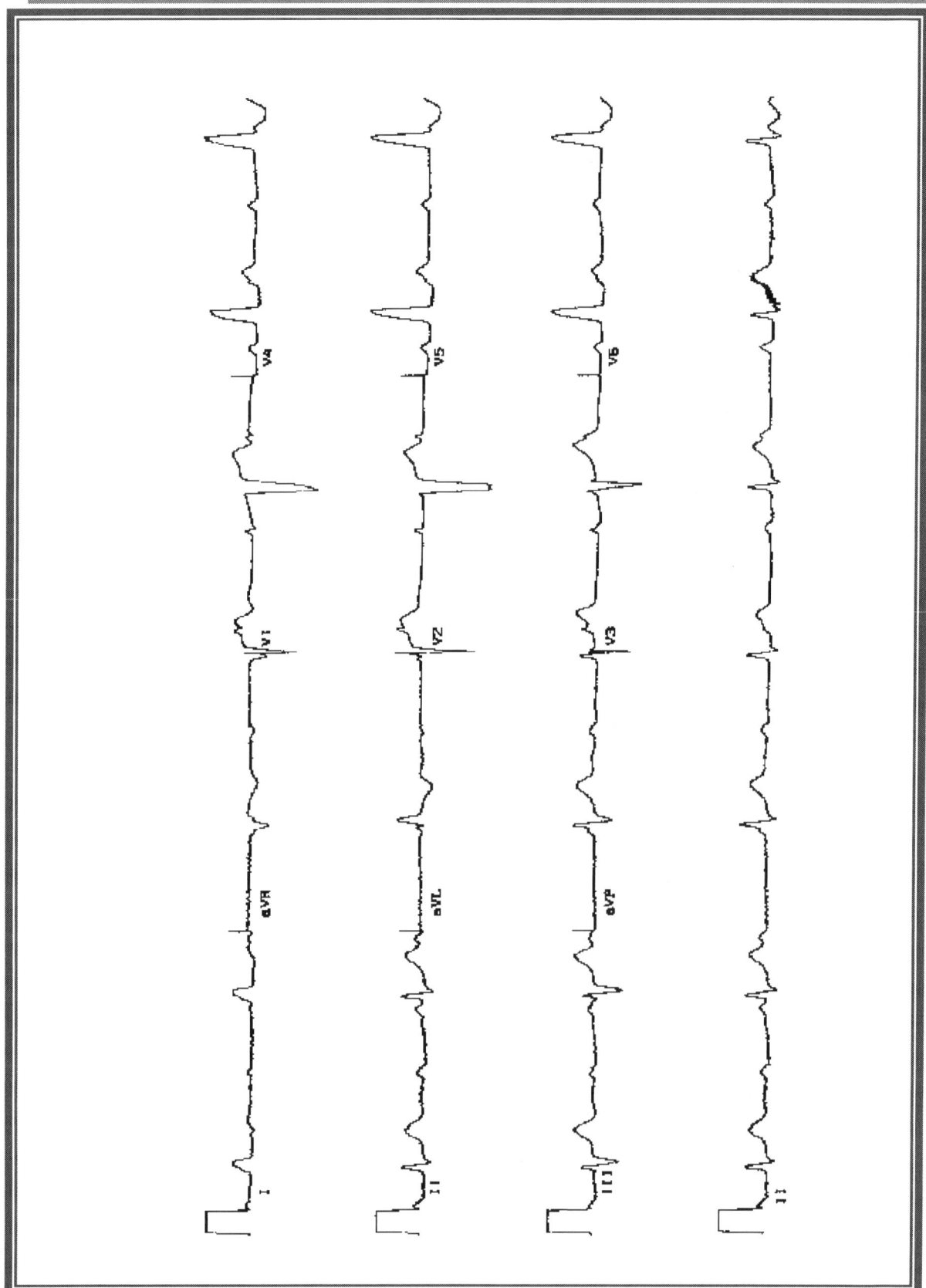

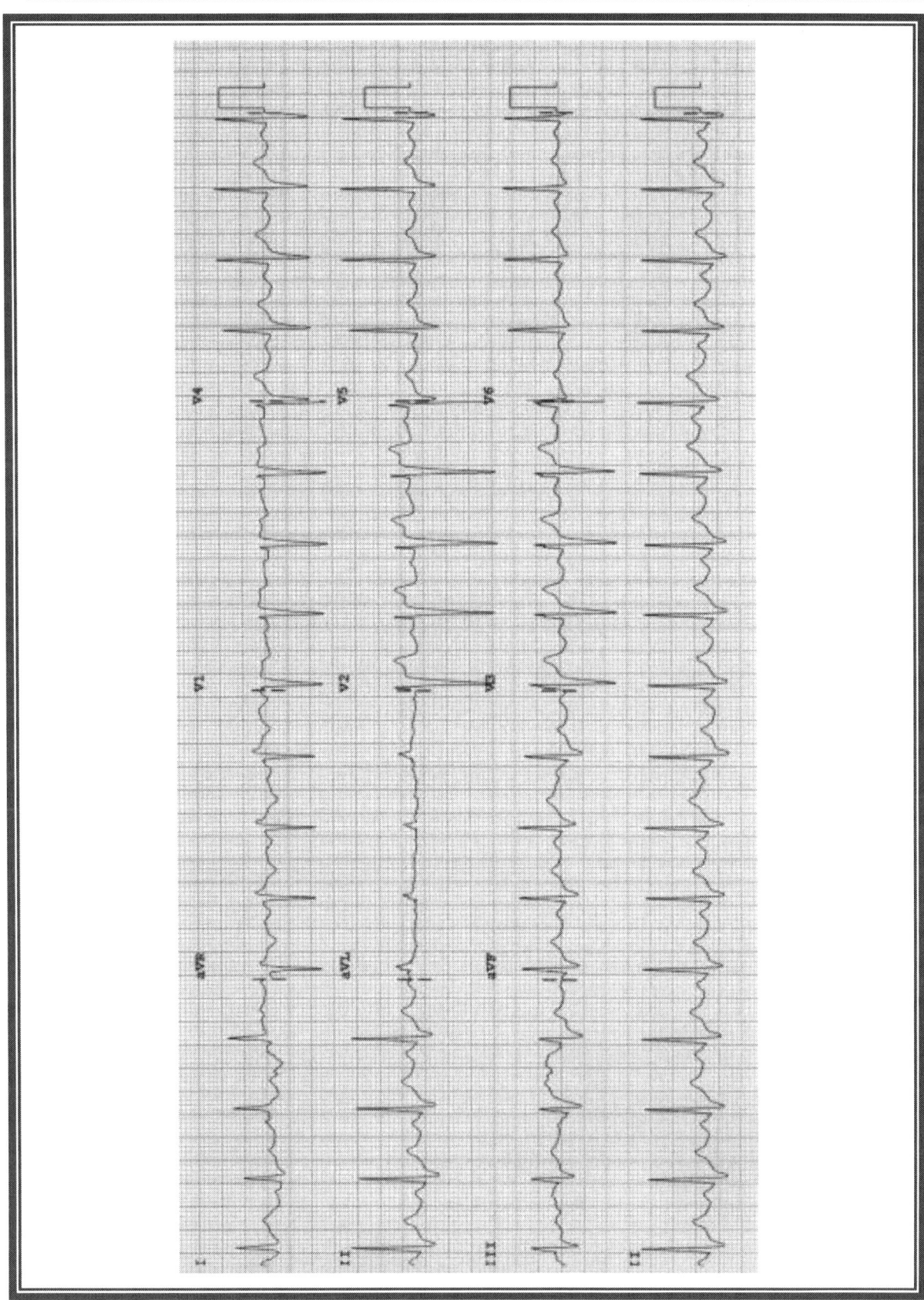

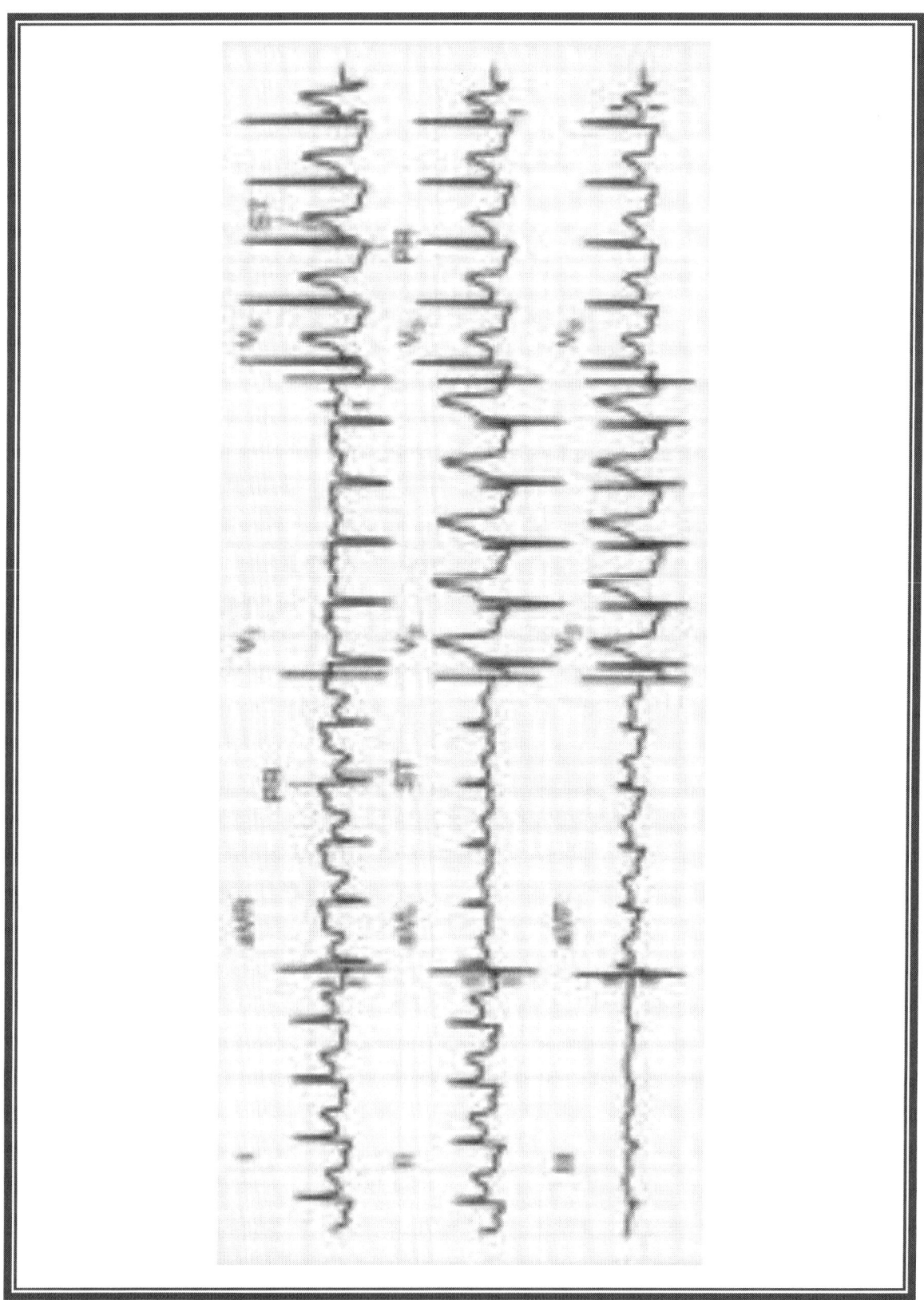

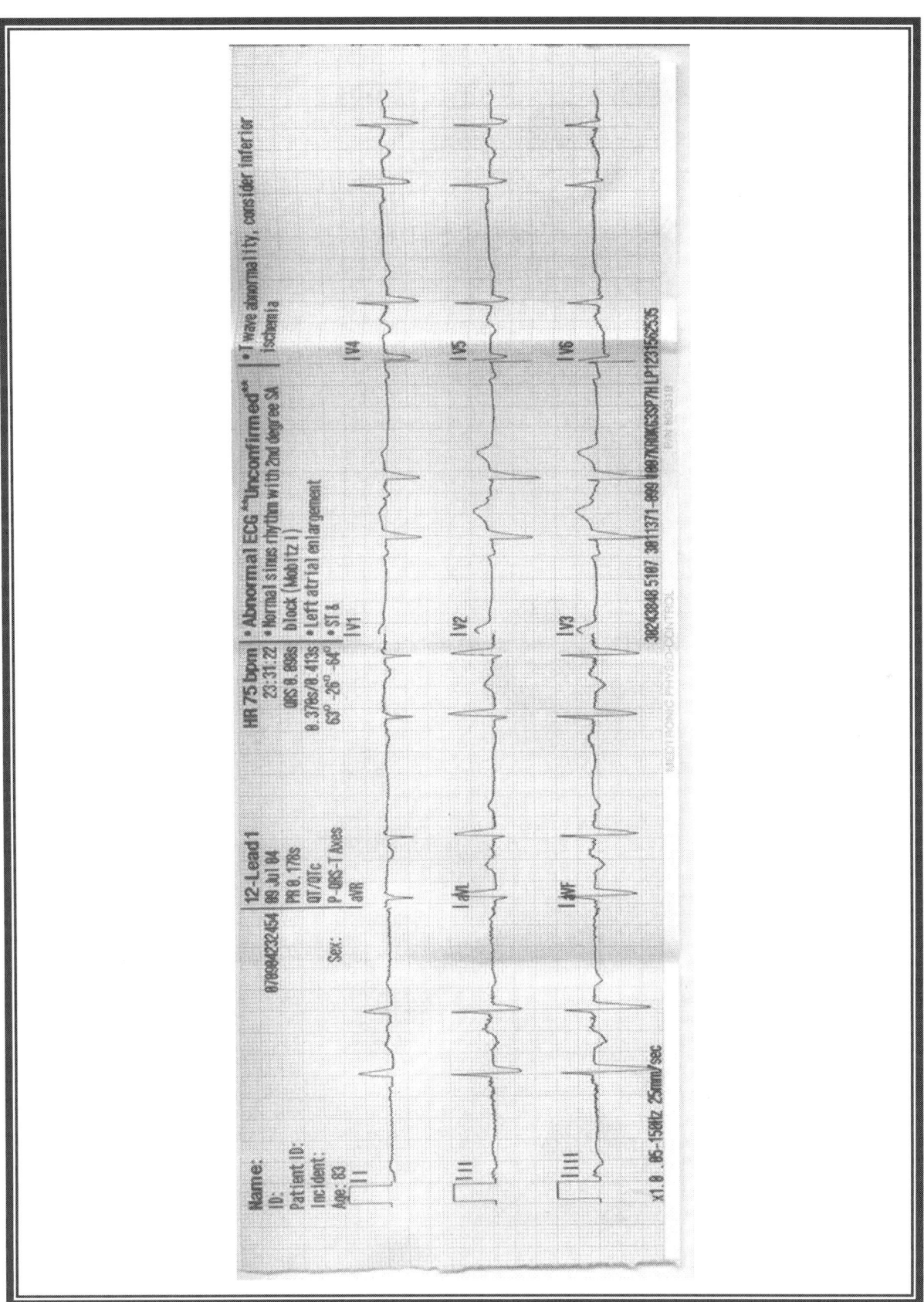

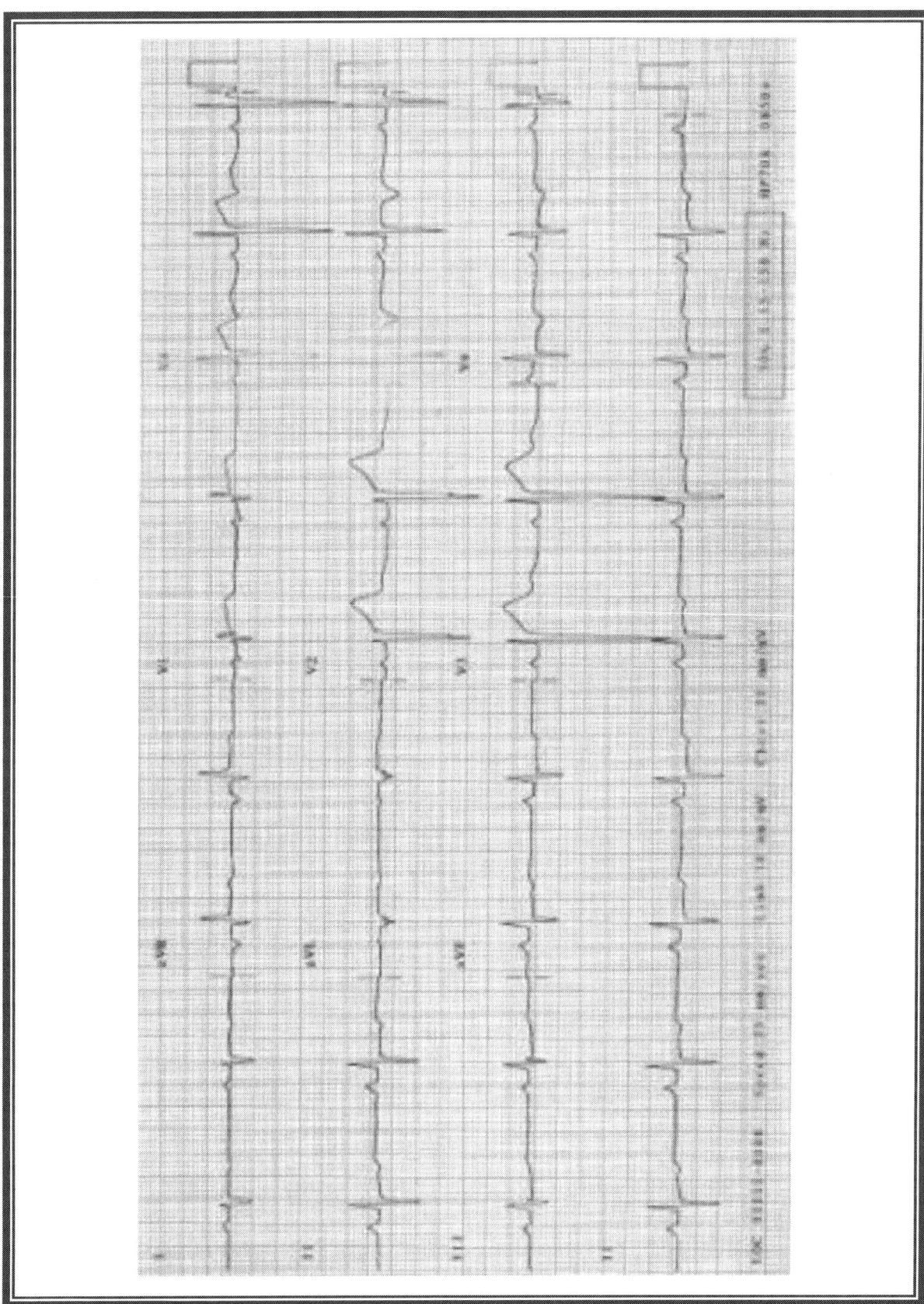

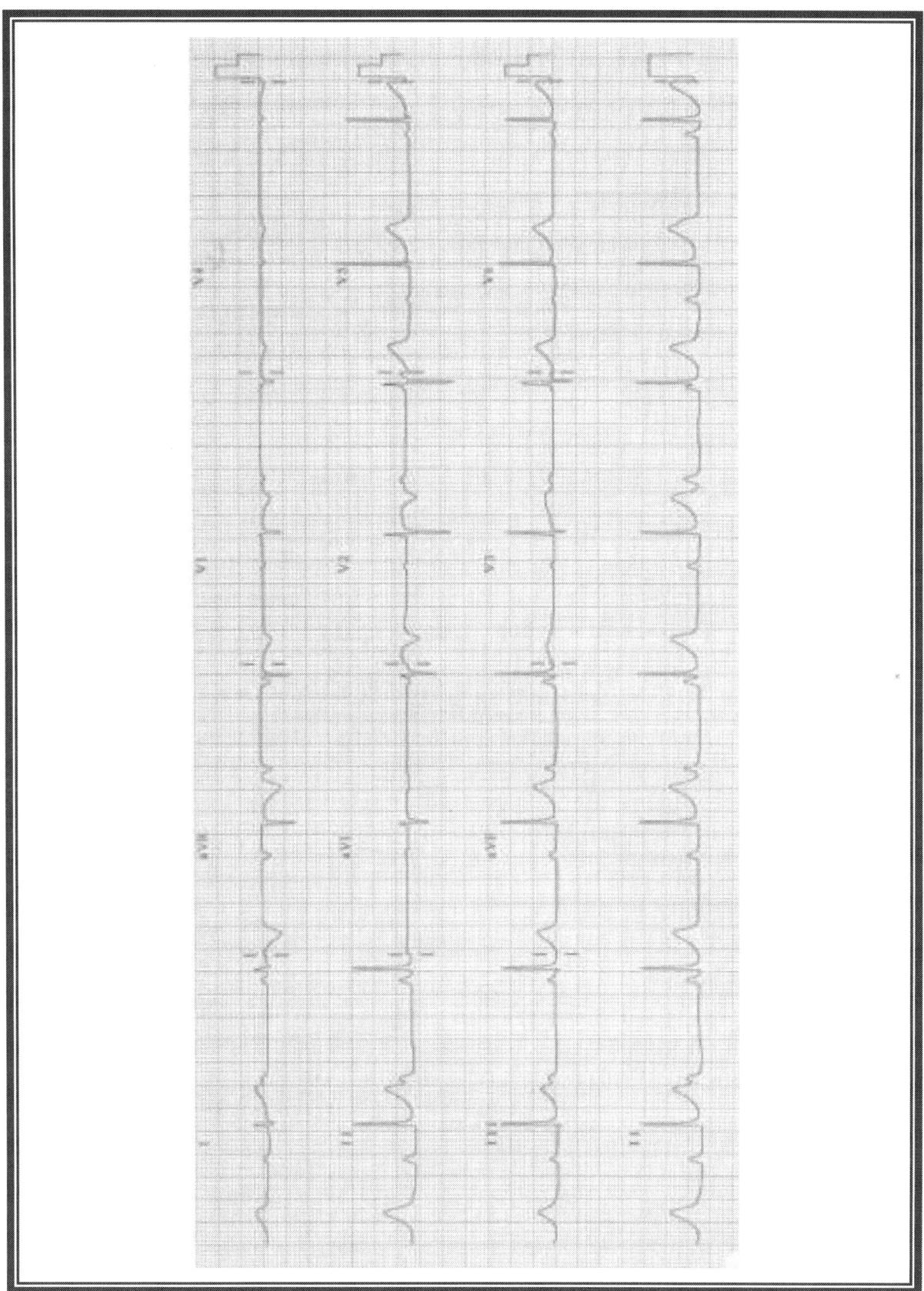

blank

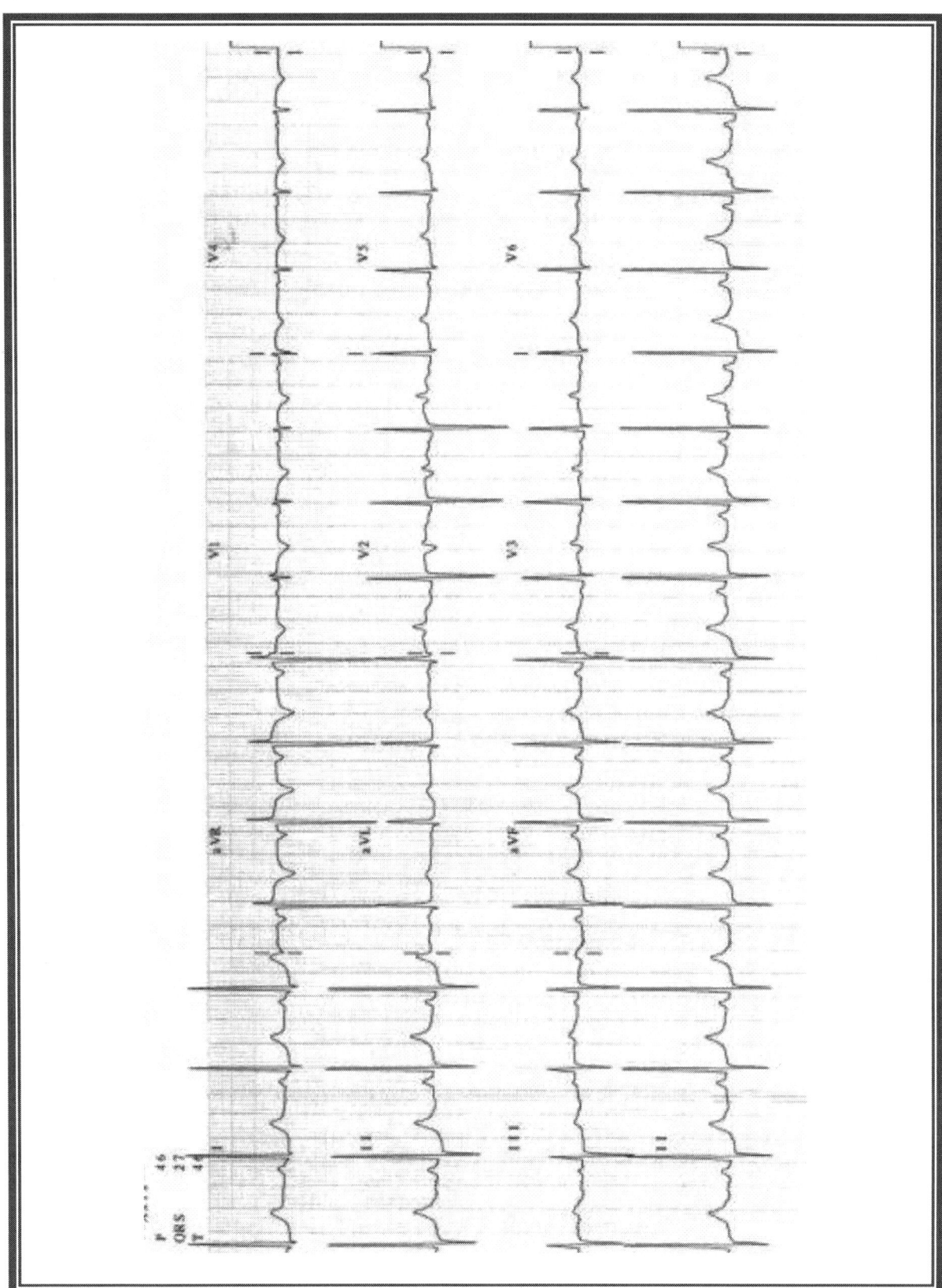

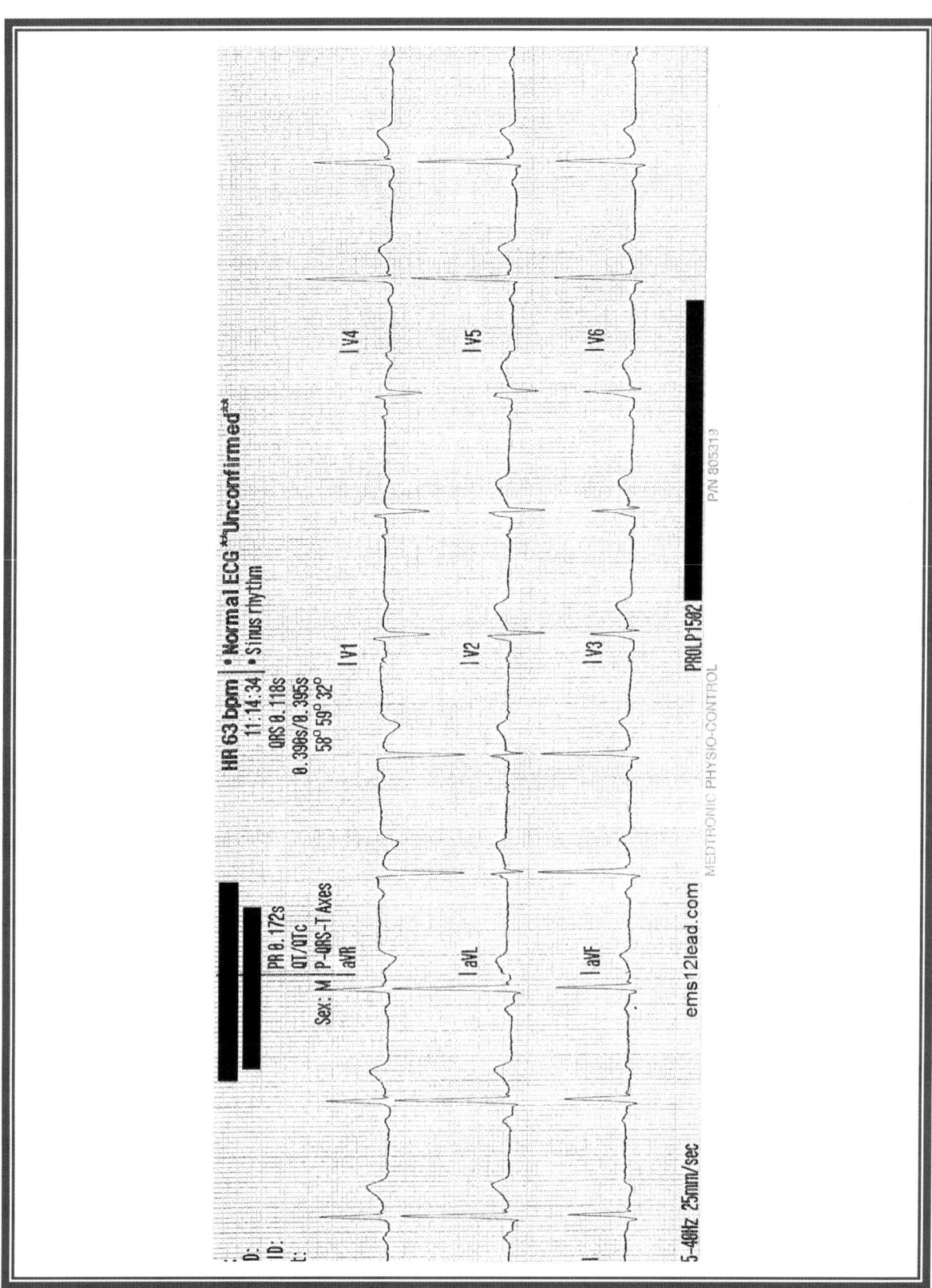

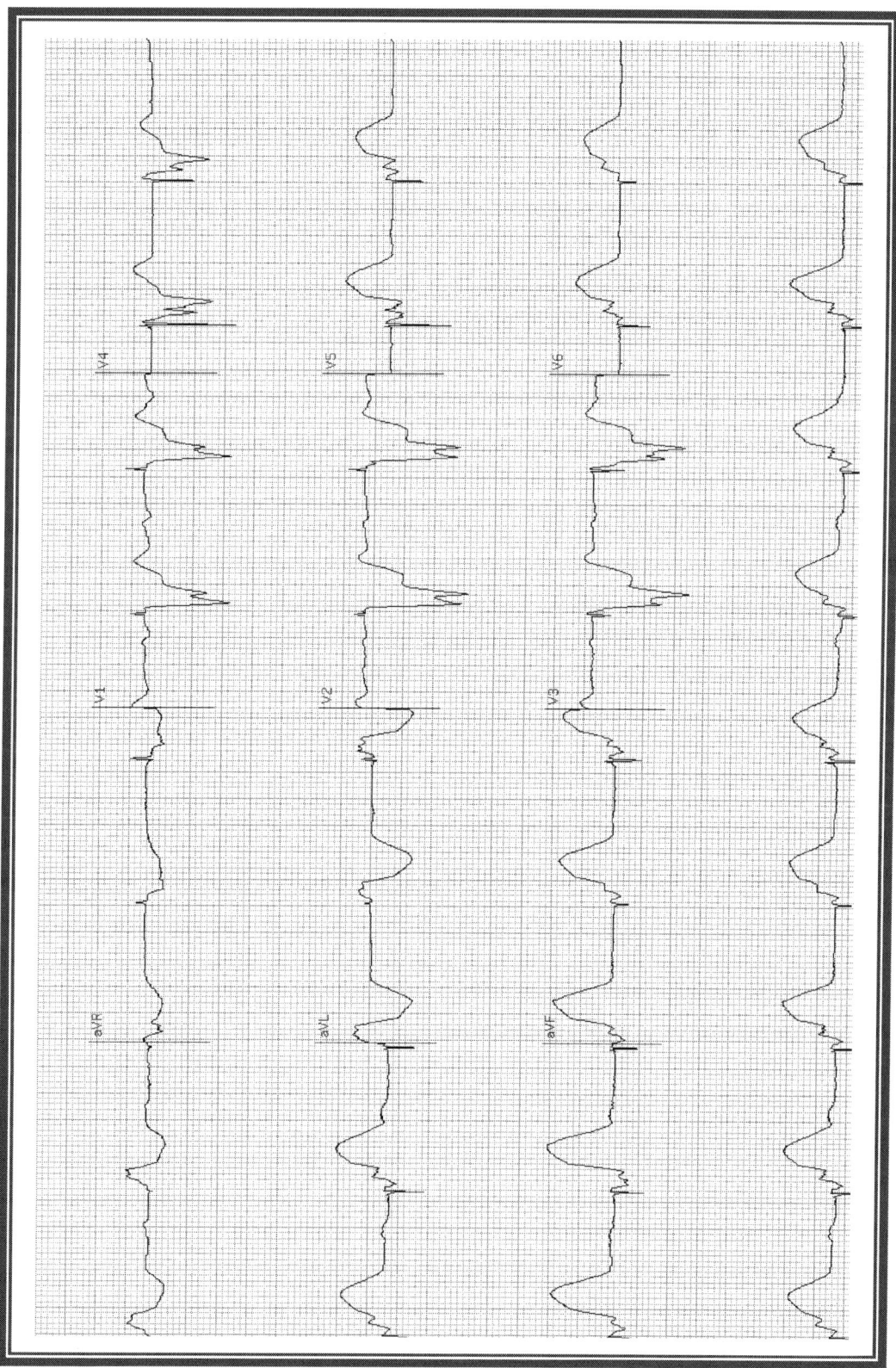

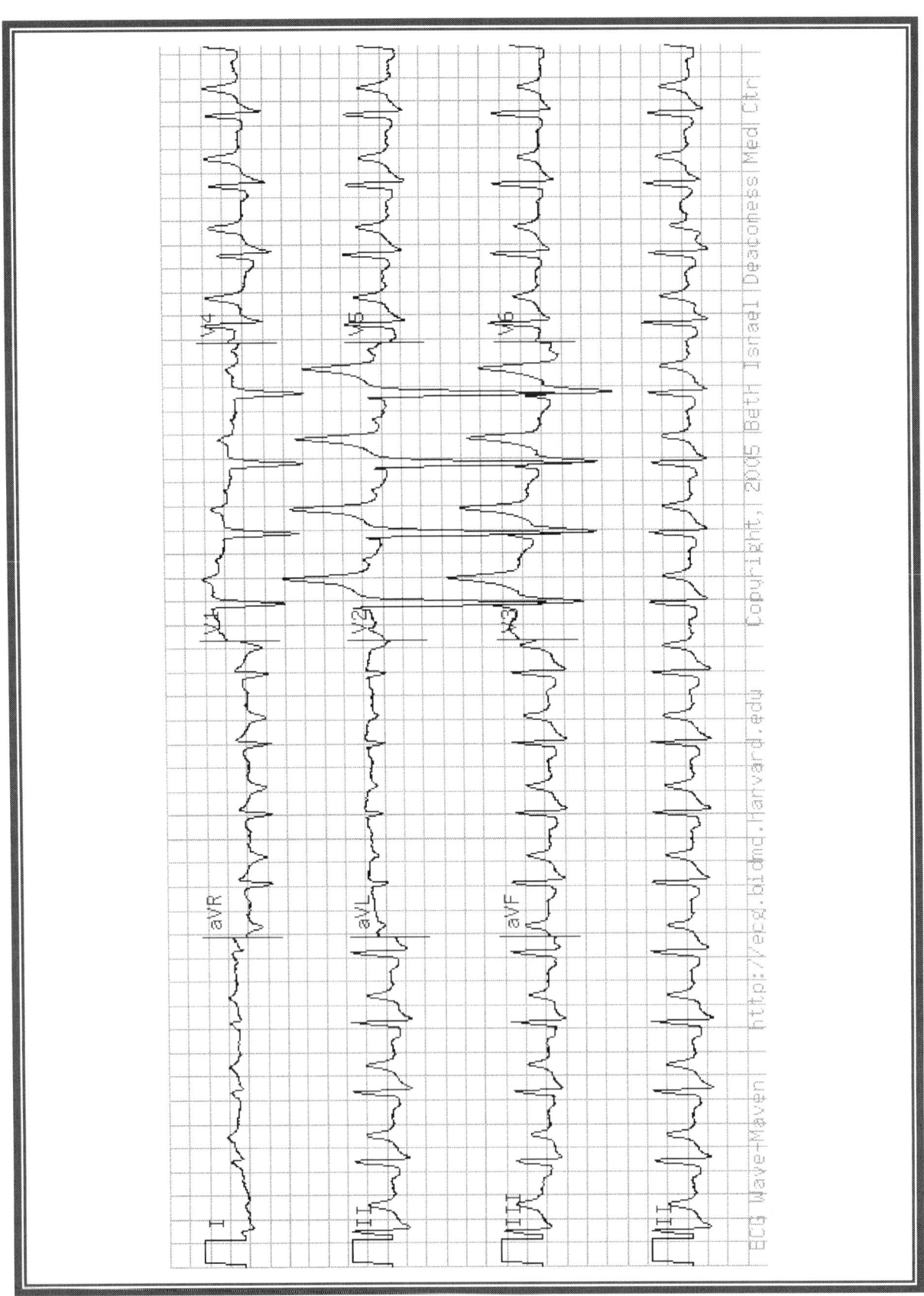

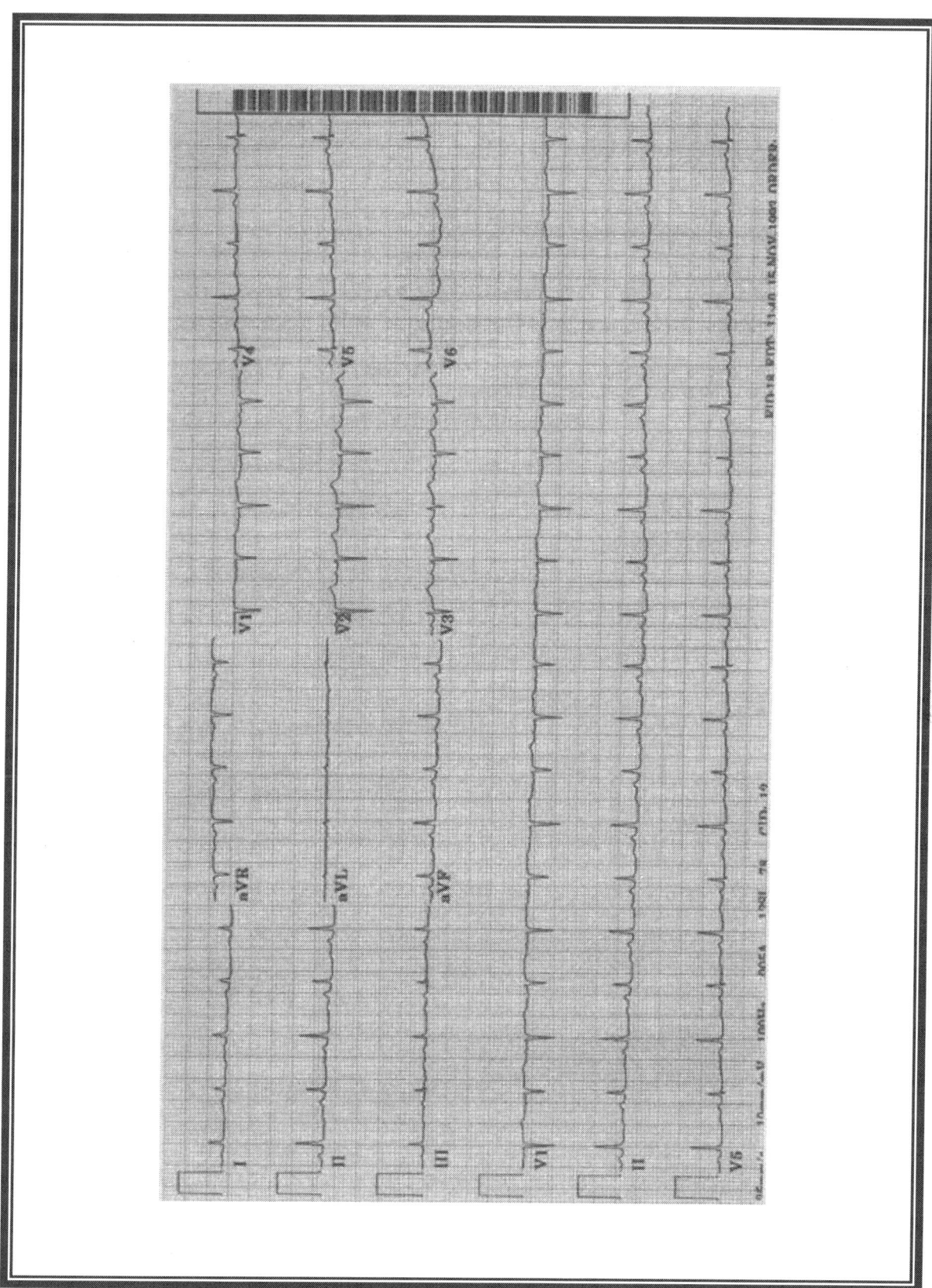

Write the Diagnosis of the previous EKG's:

1._____

2._____

3._____

4._____

5._____

6._____

7._____

8._____

9._____

10._____

11._____

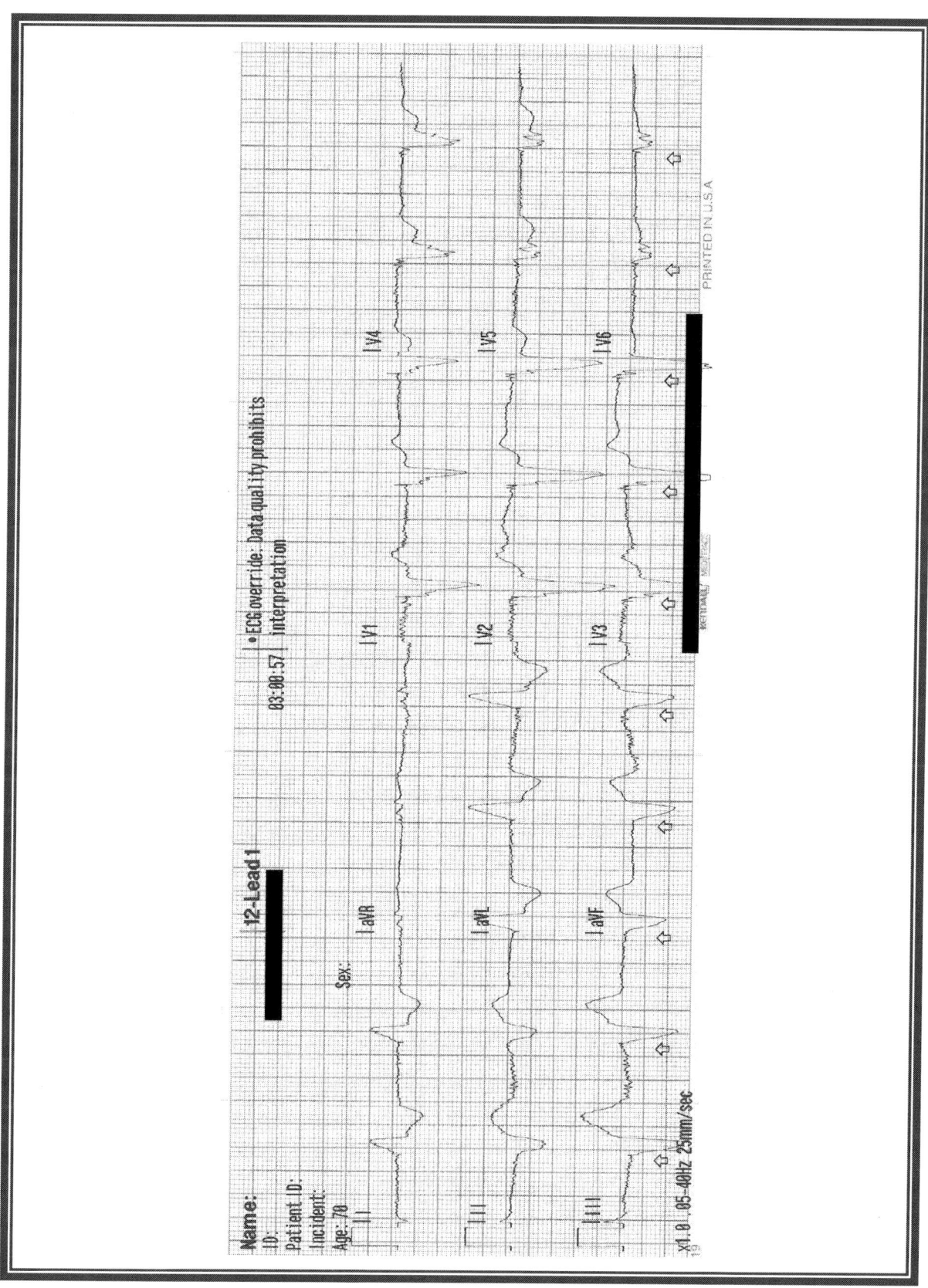

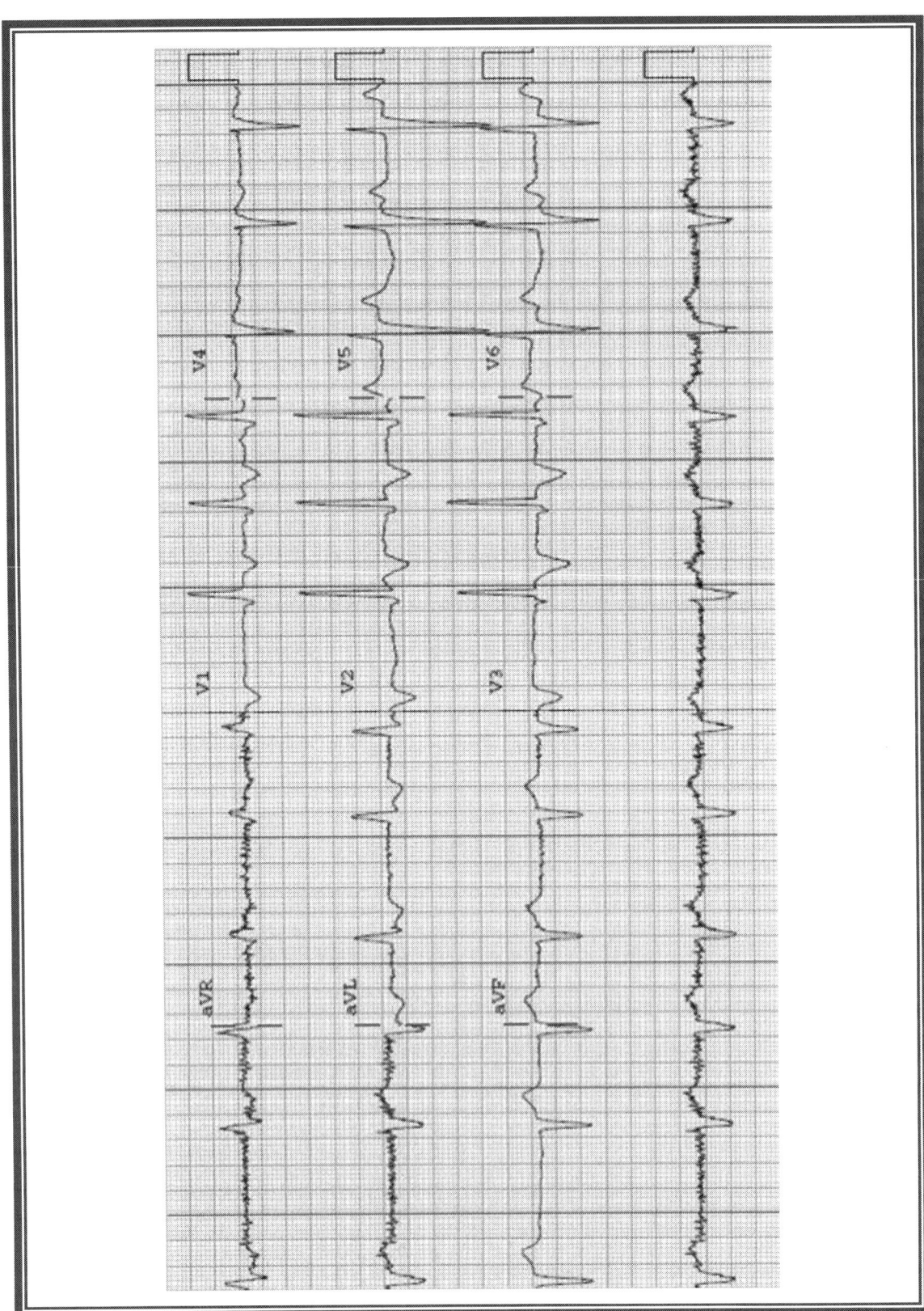

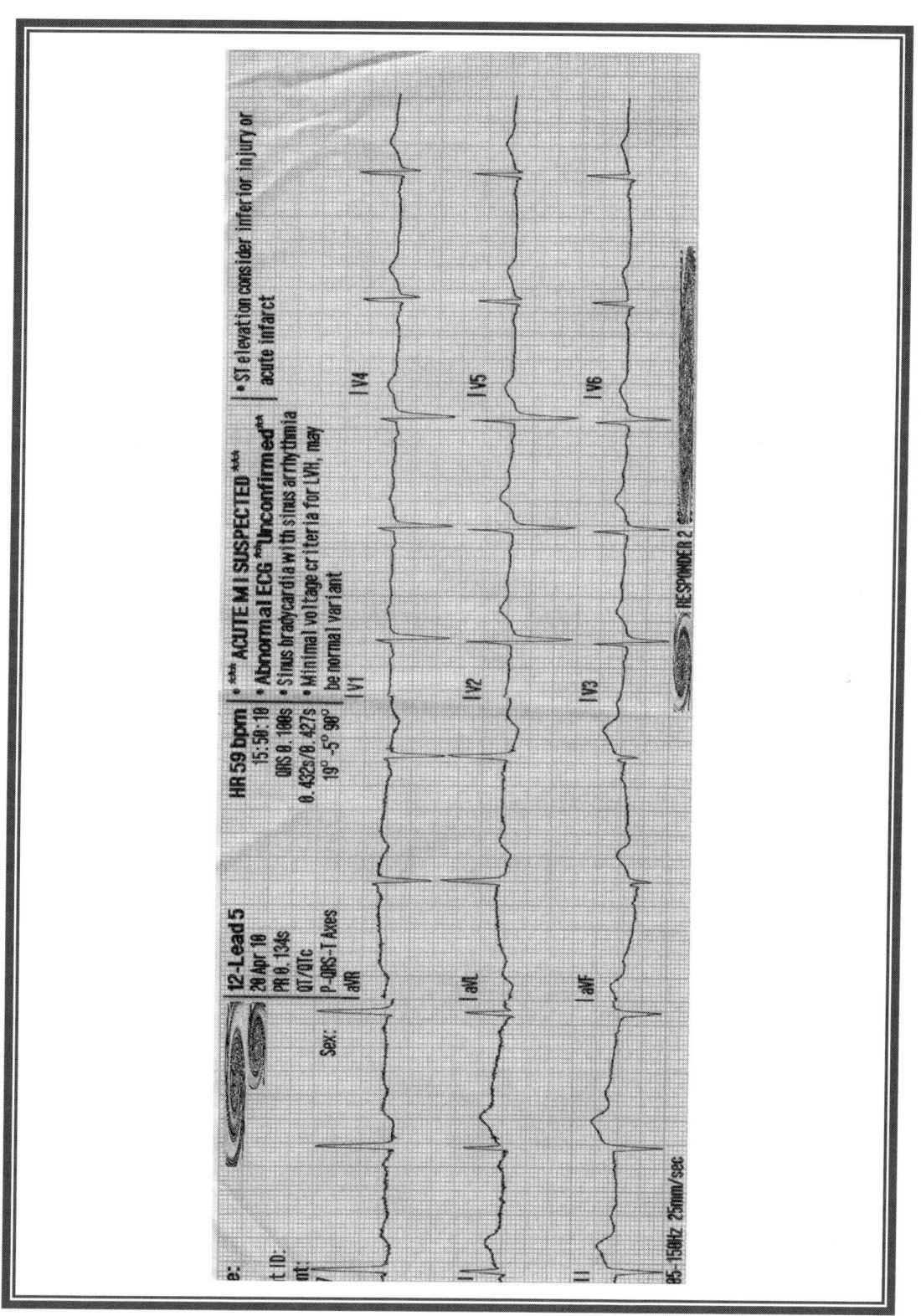

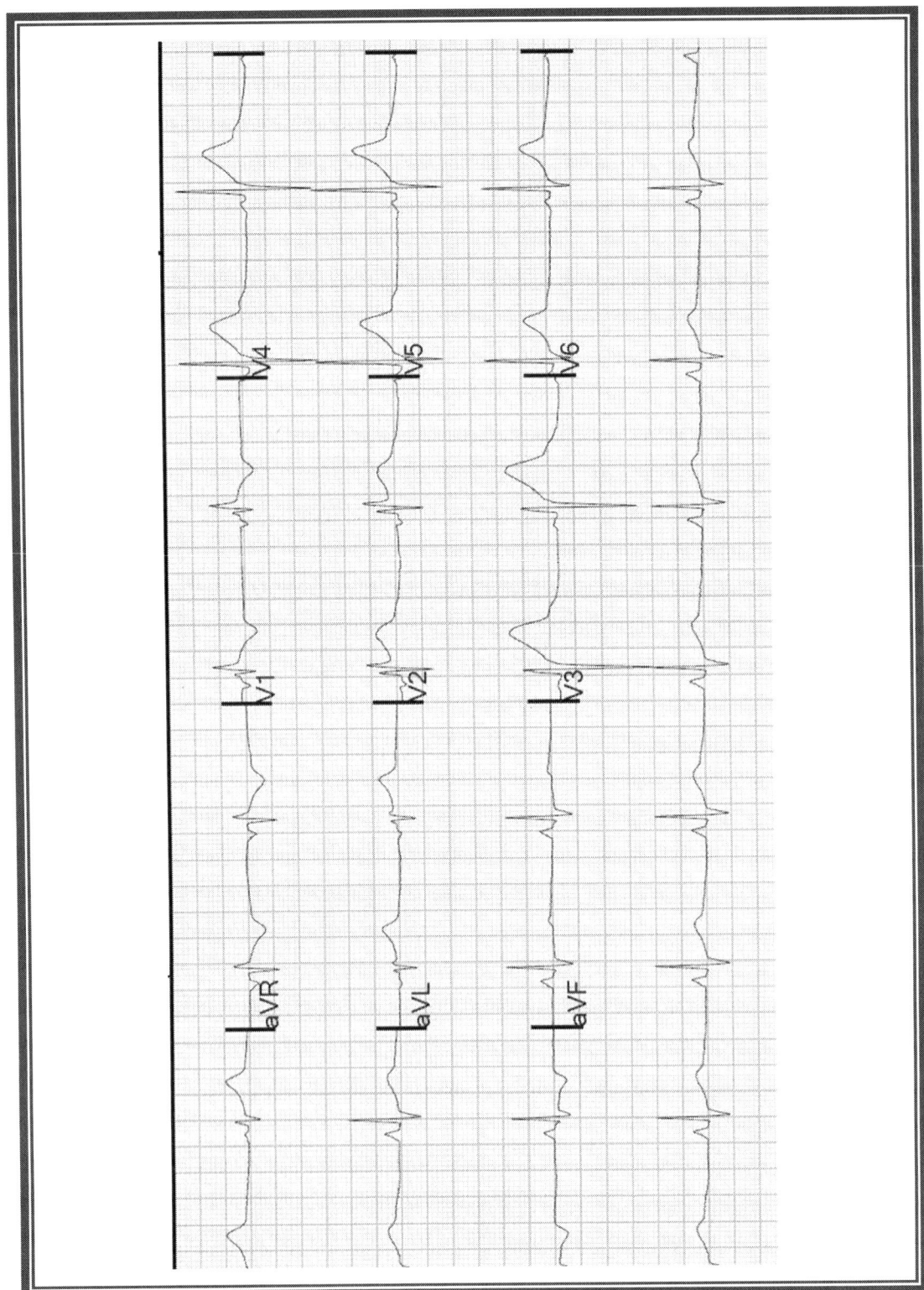

Write the Diagnosis of the previous EKG's:

1._____

2._____

3._____

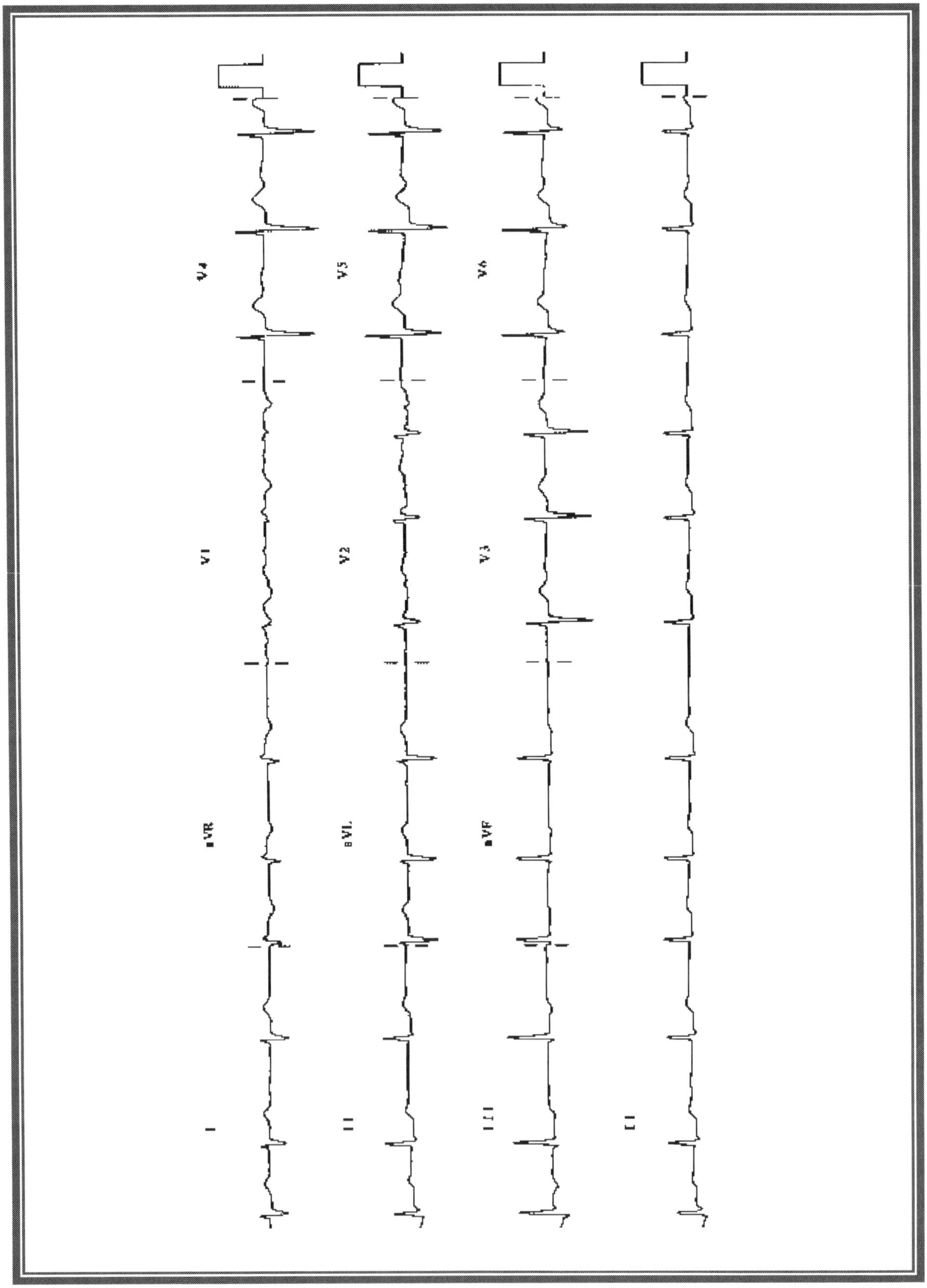
I
aVR
V1
V4
II
aVL
V2
V5
III
aVF
V3
V6
II

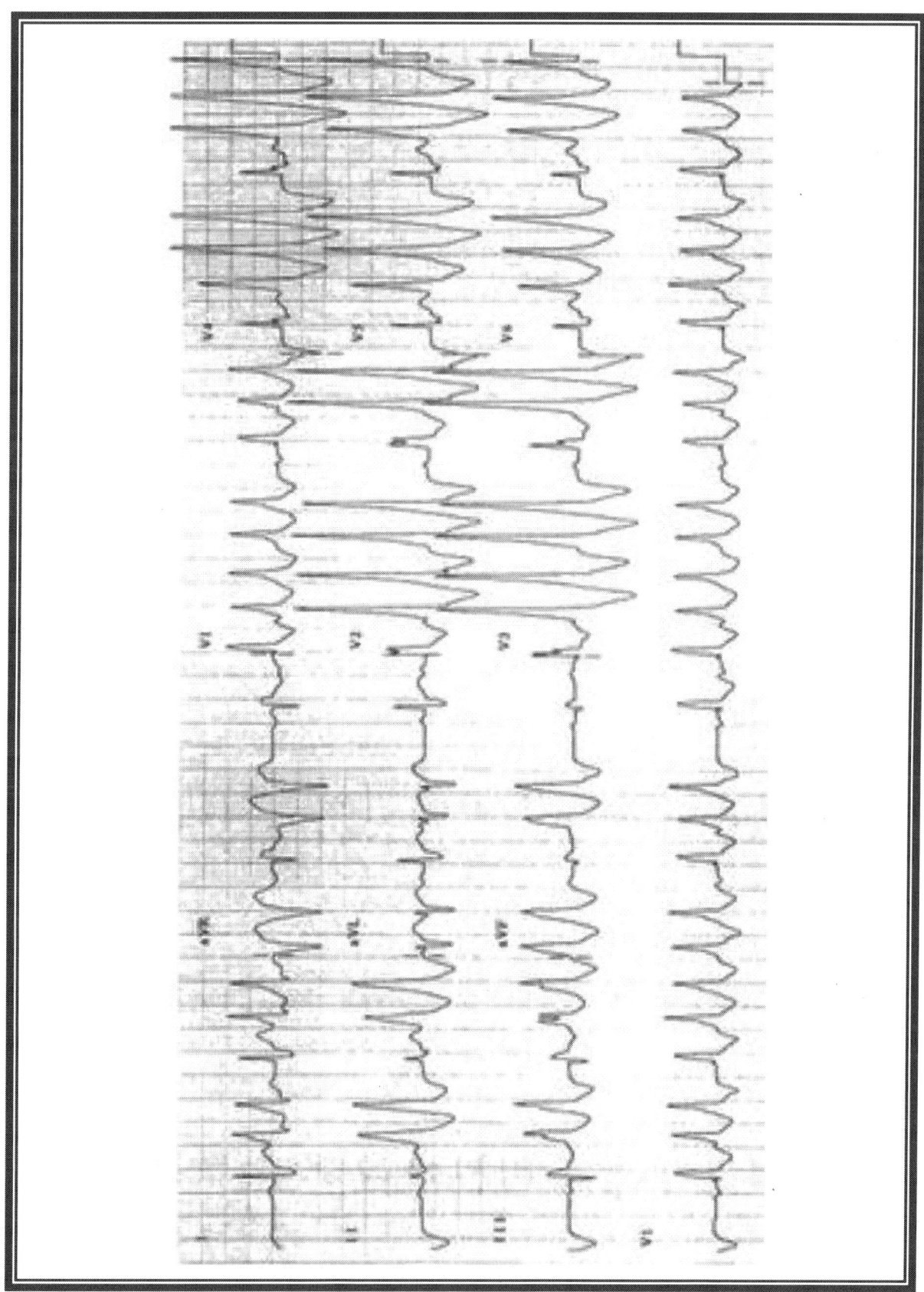

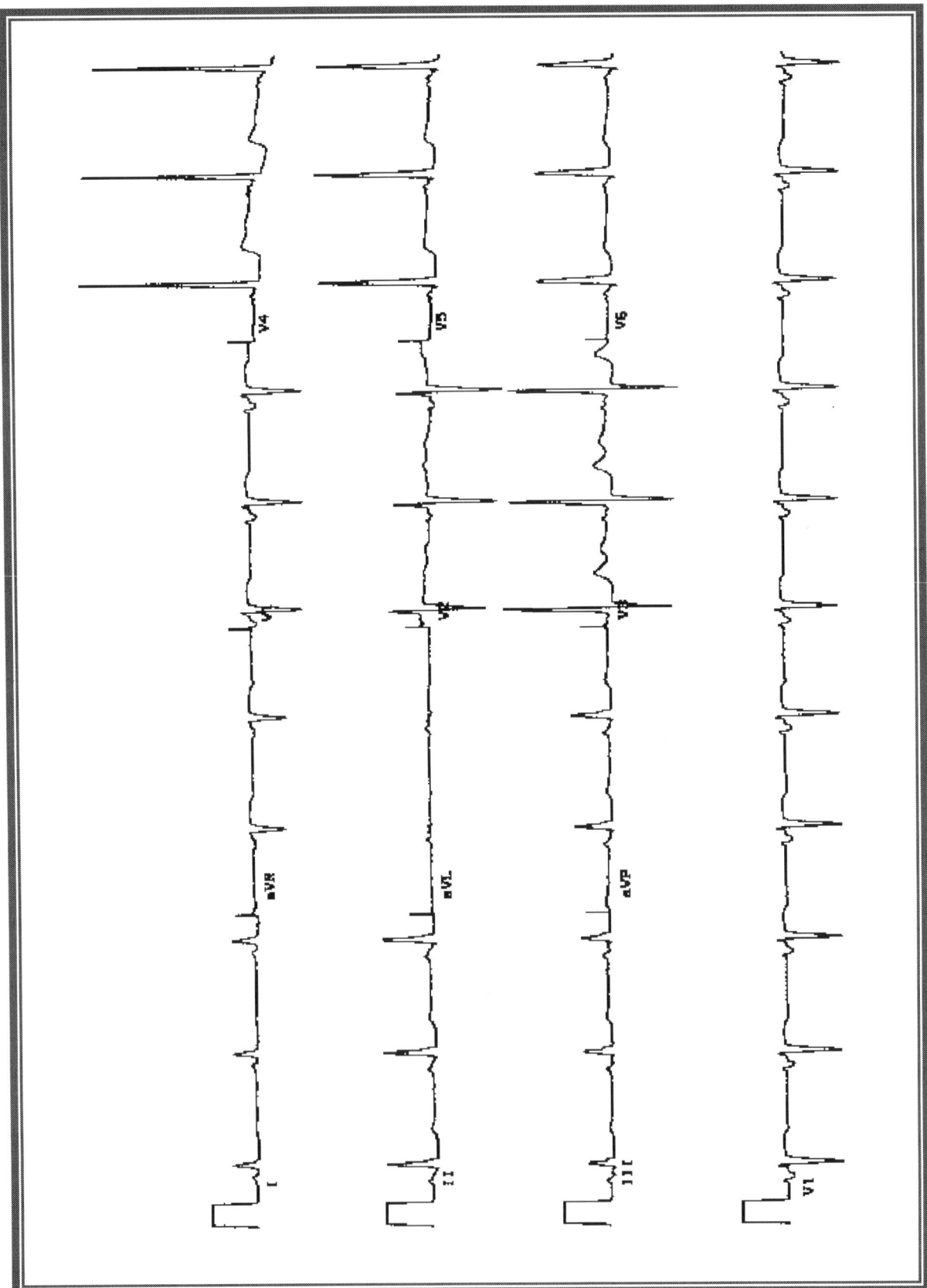

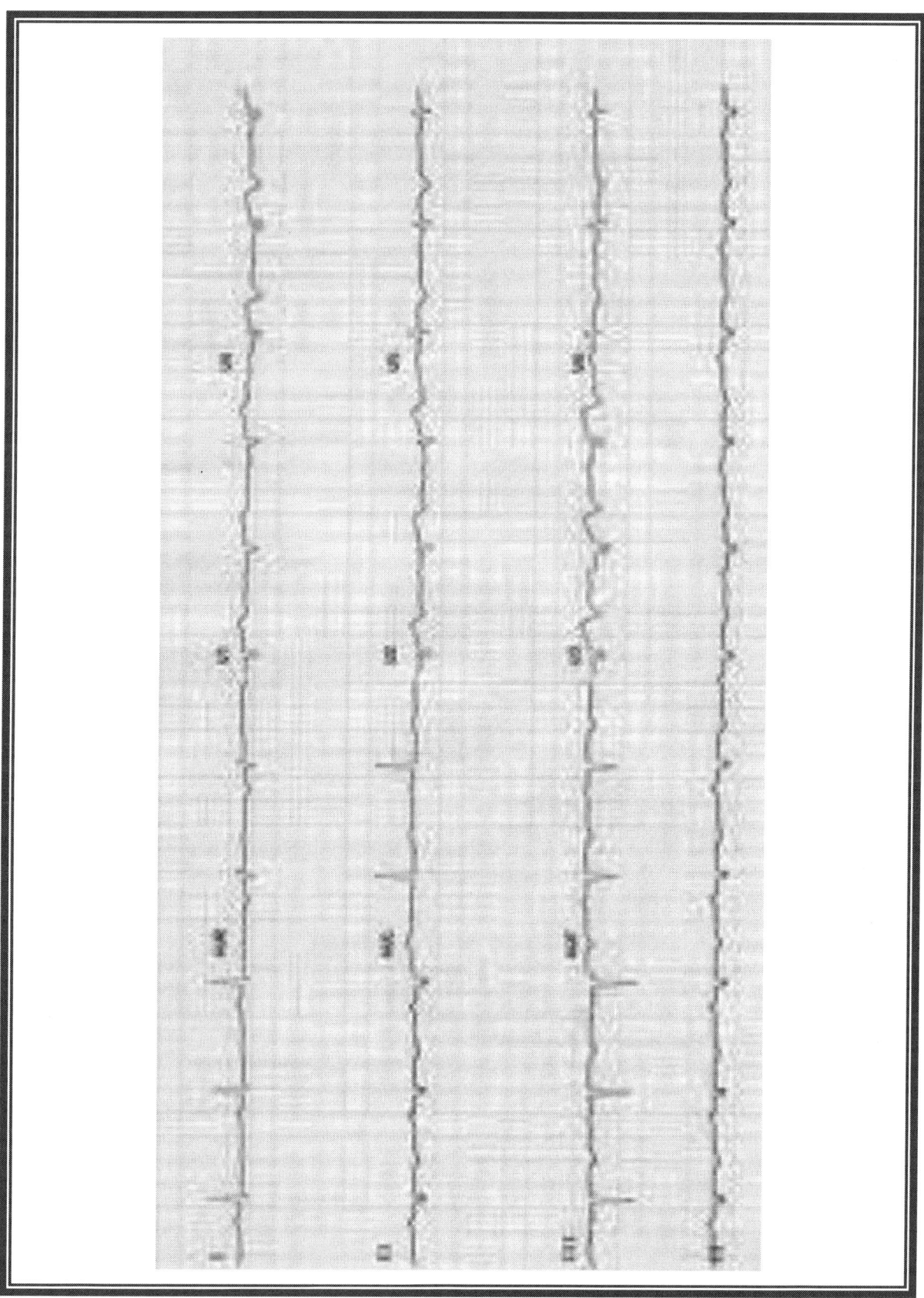

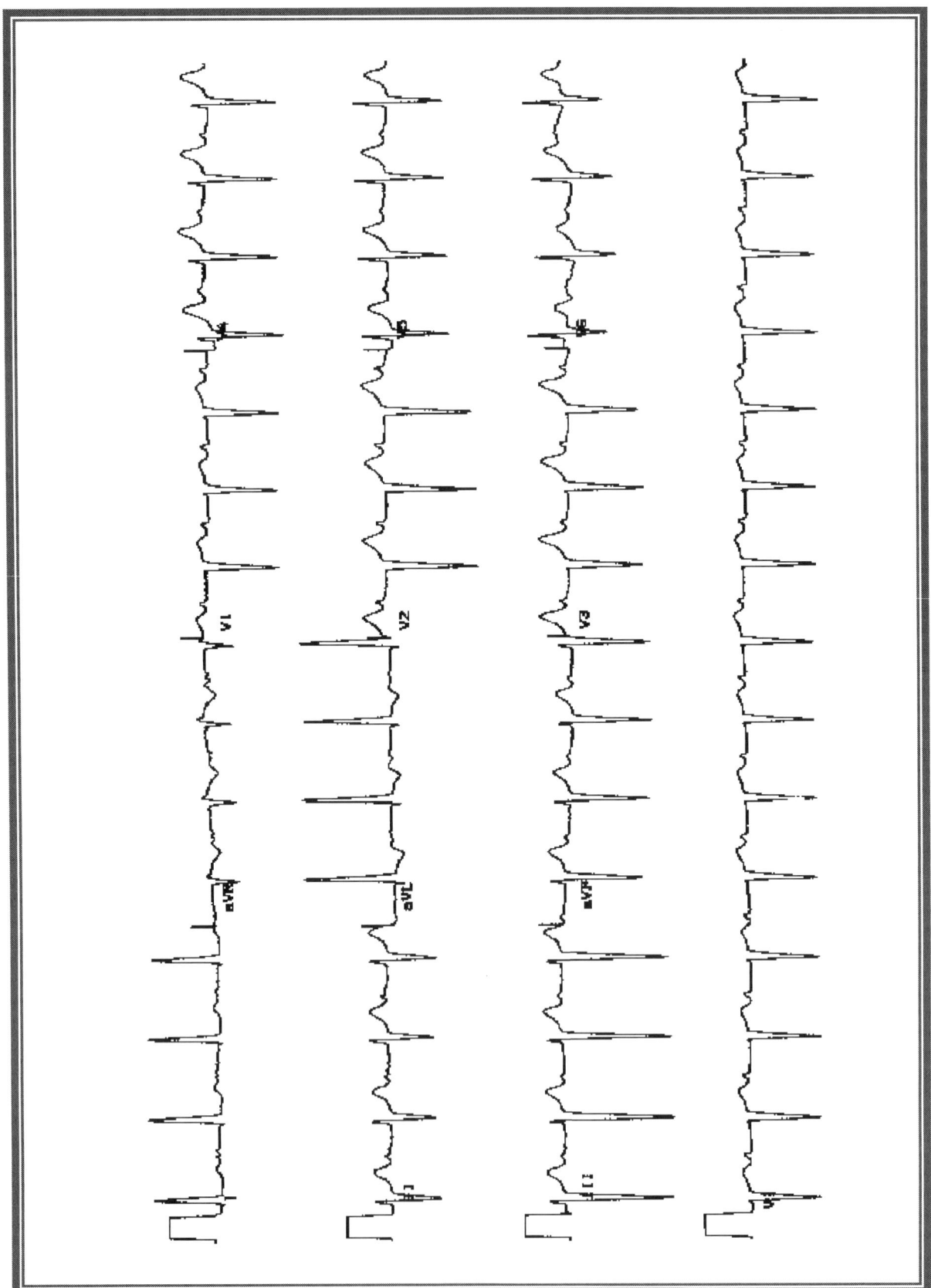

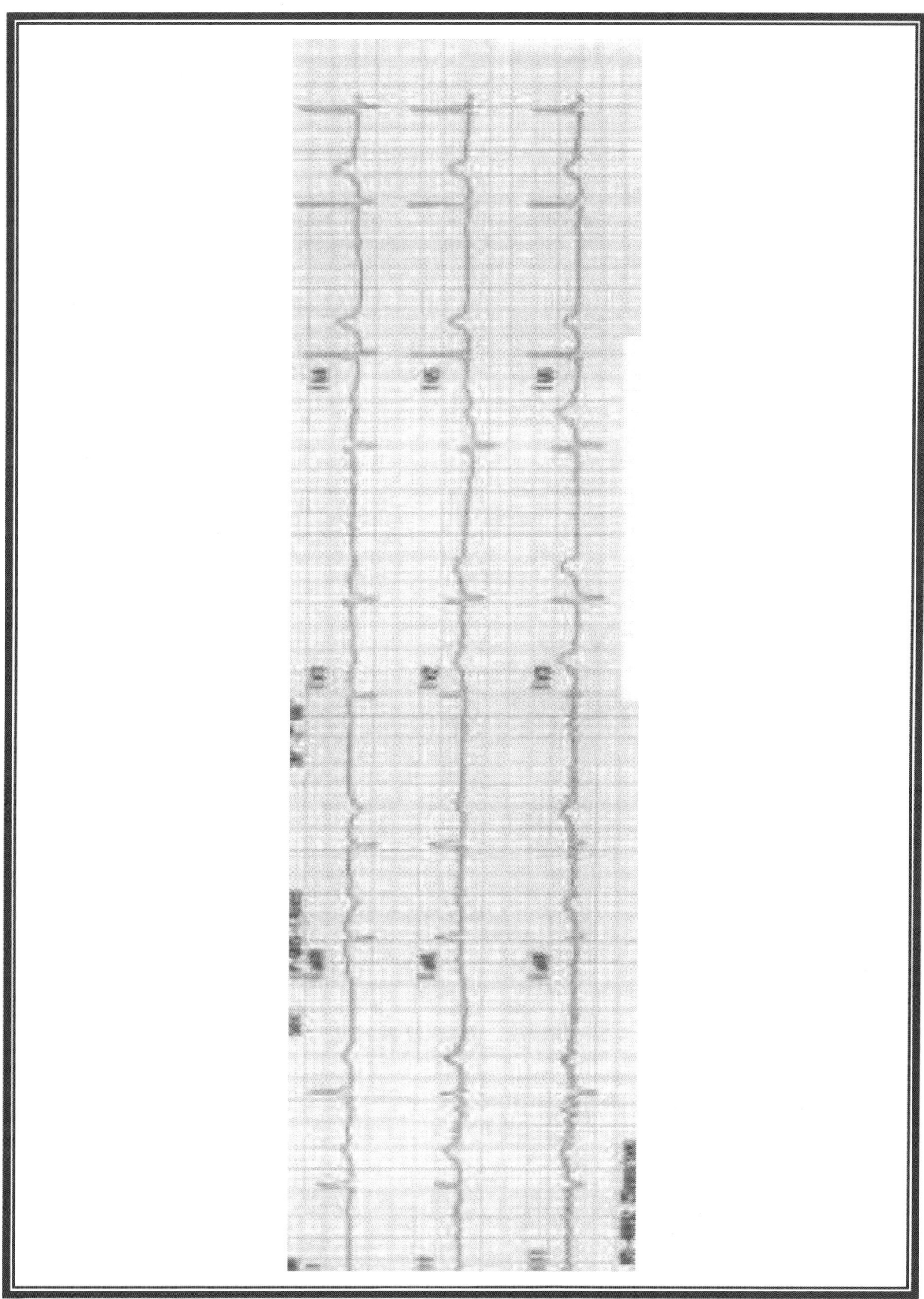

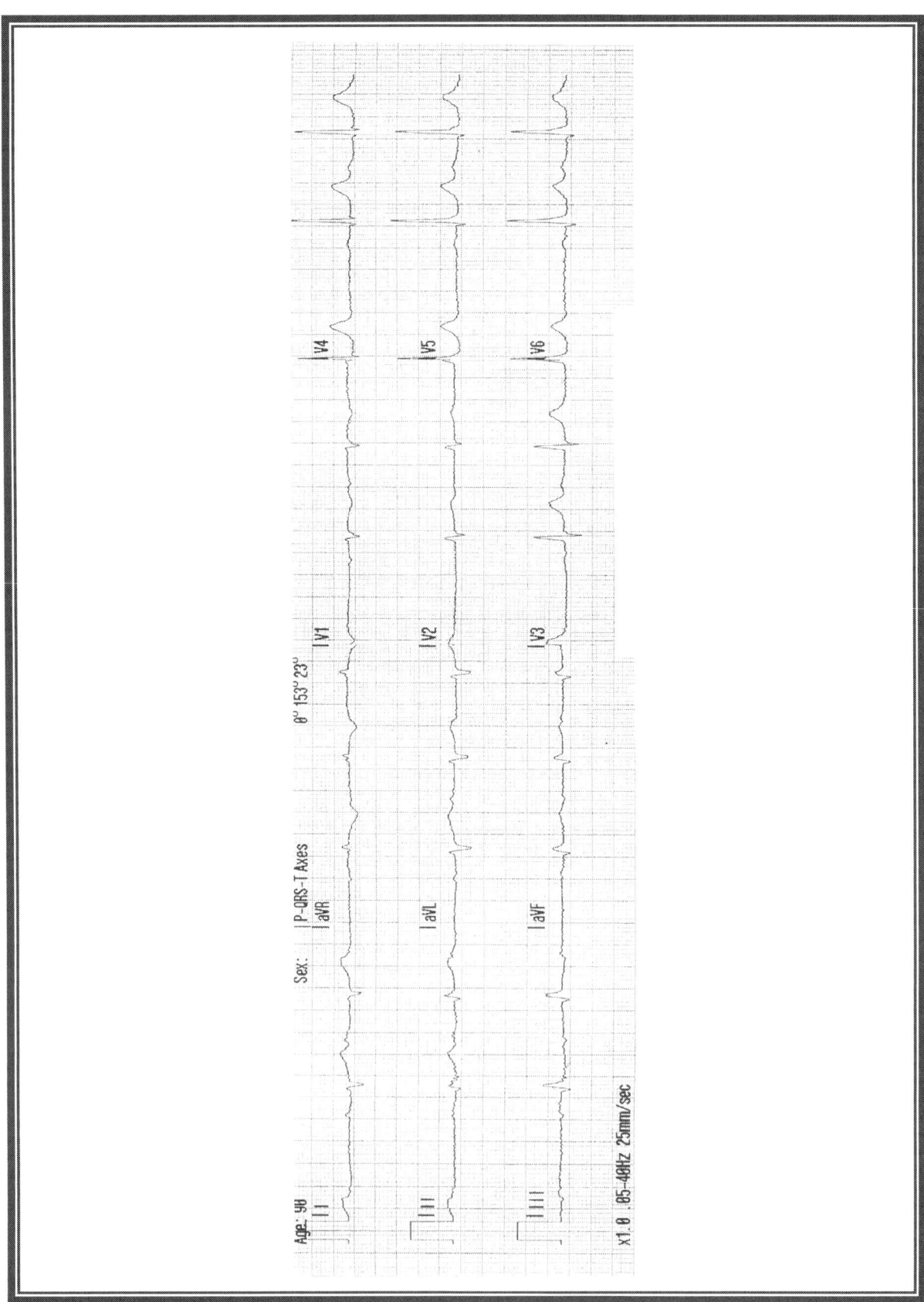

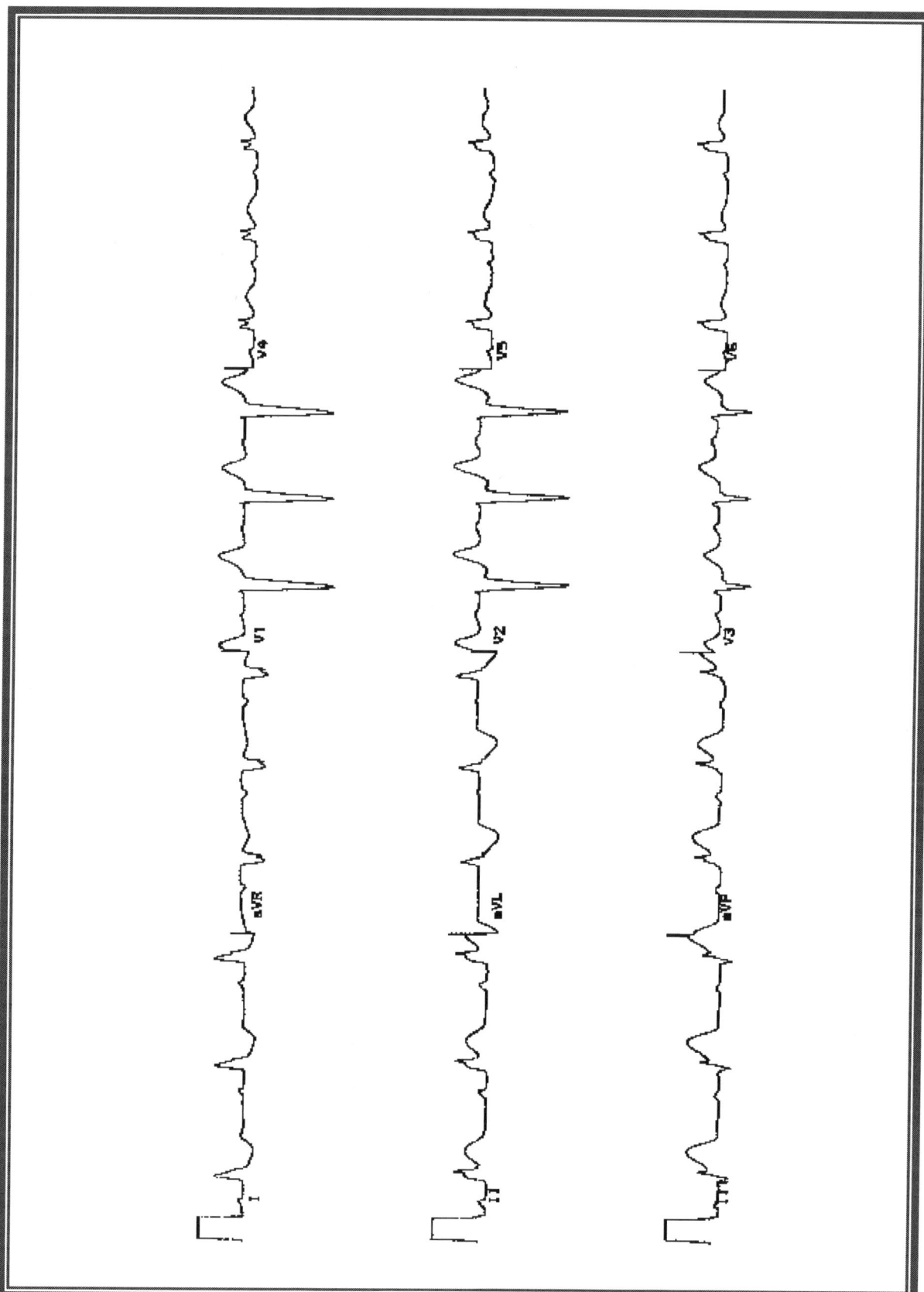

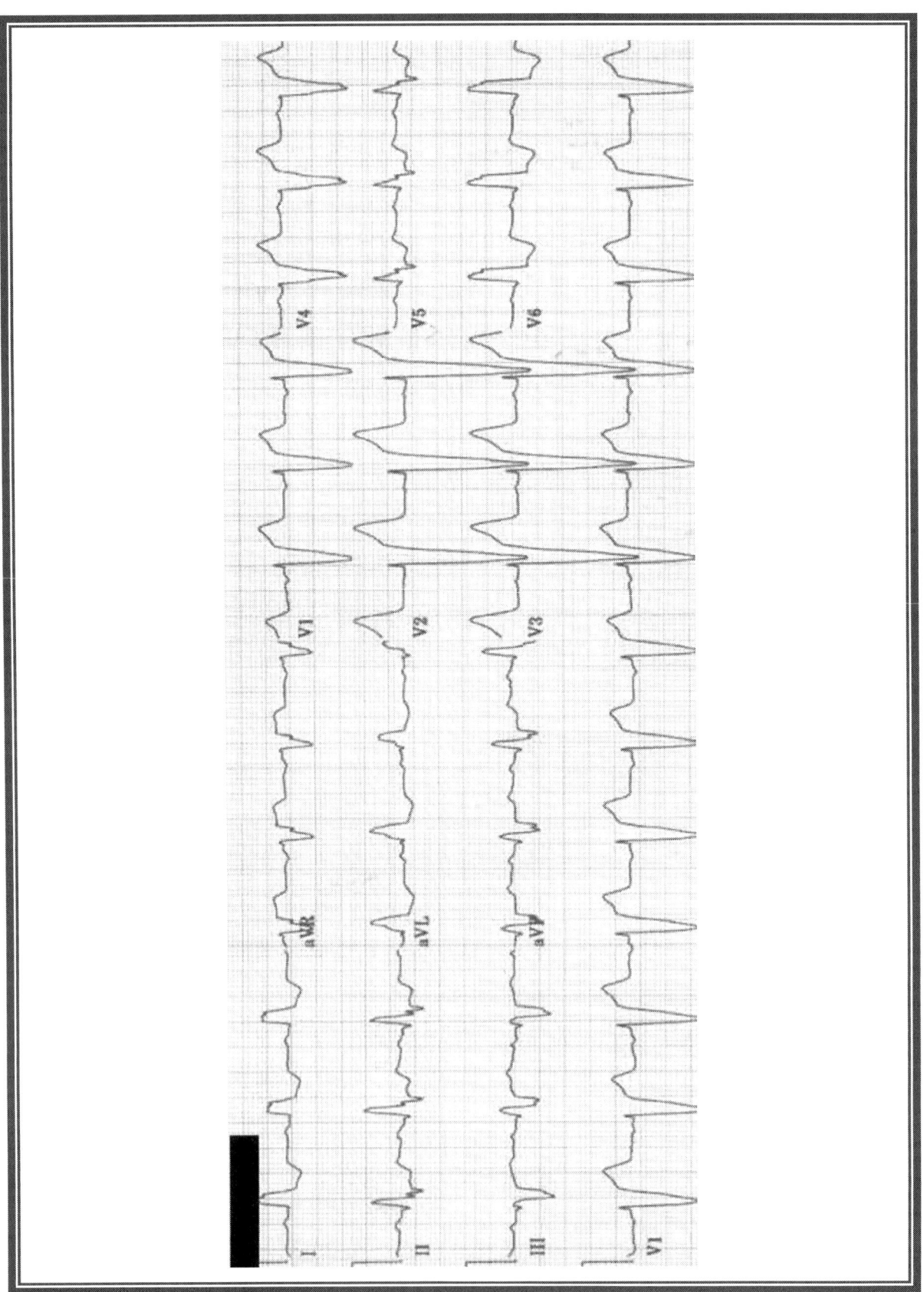

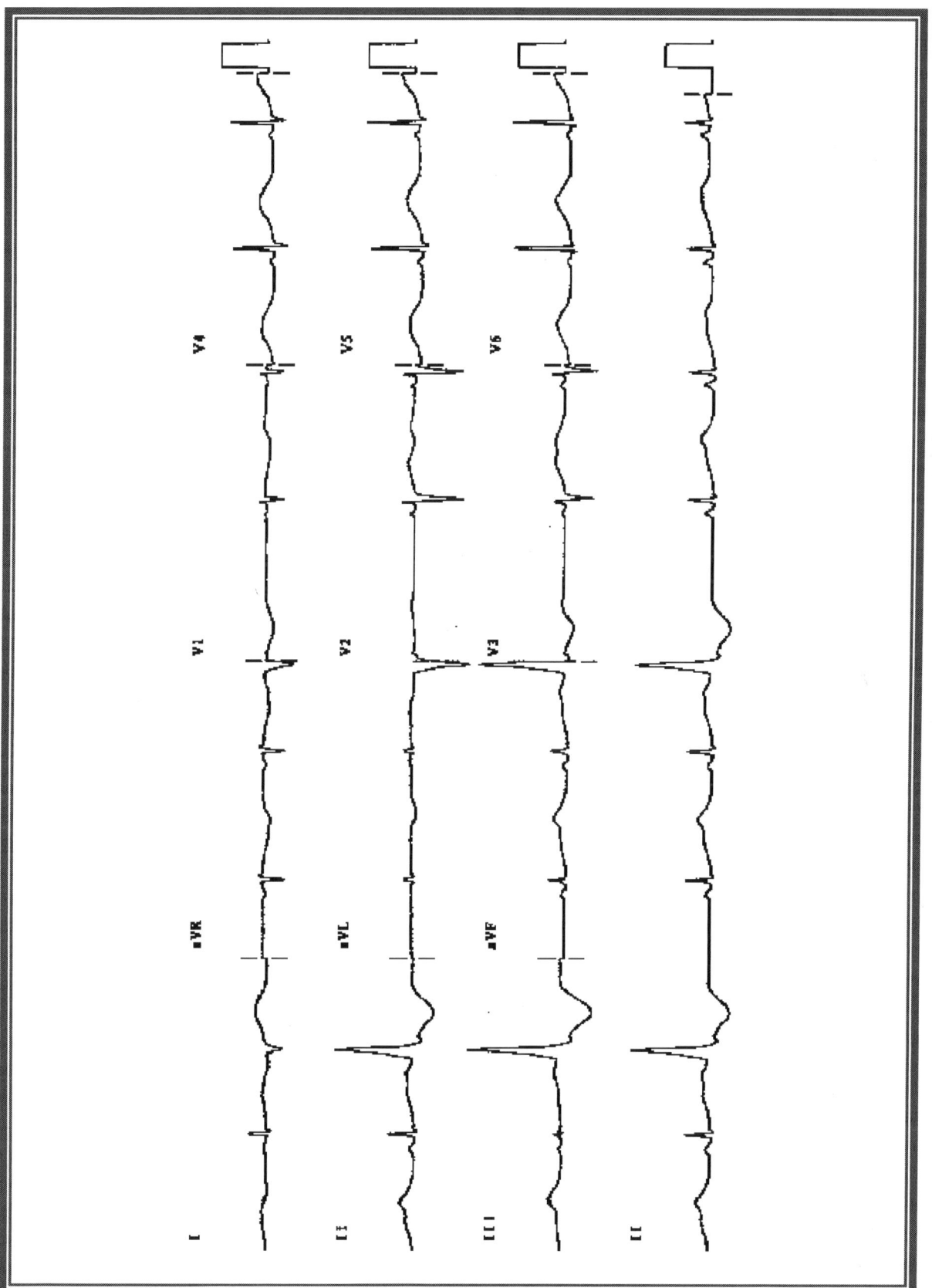

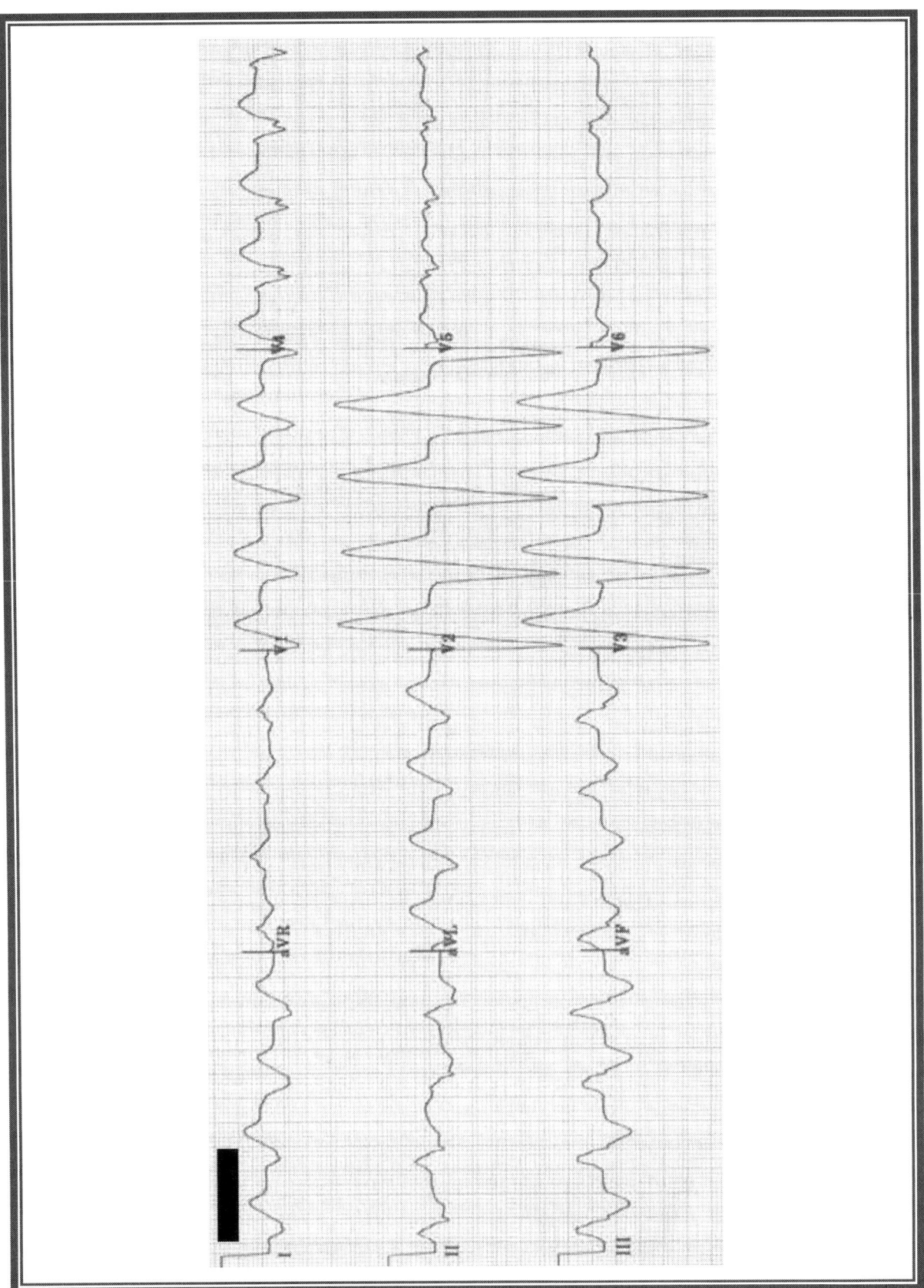

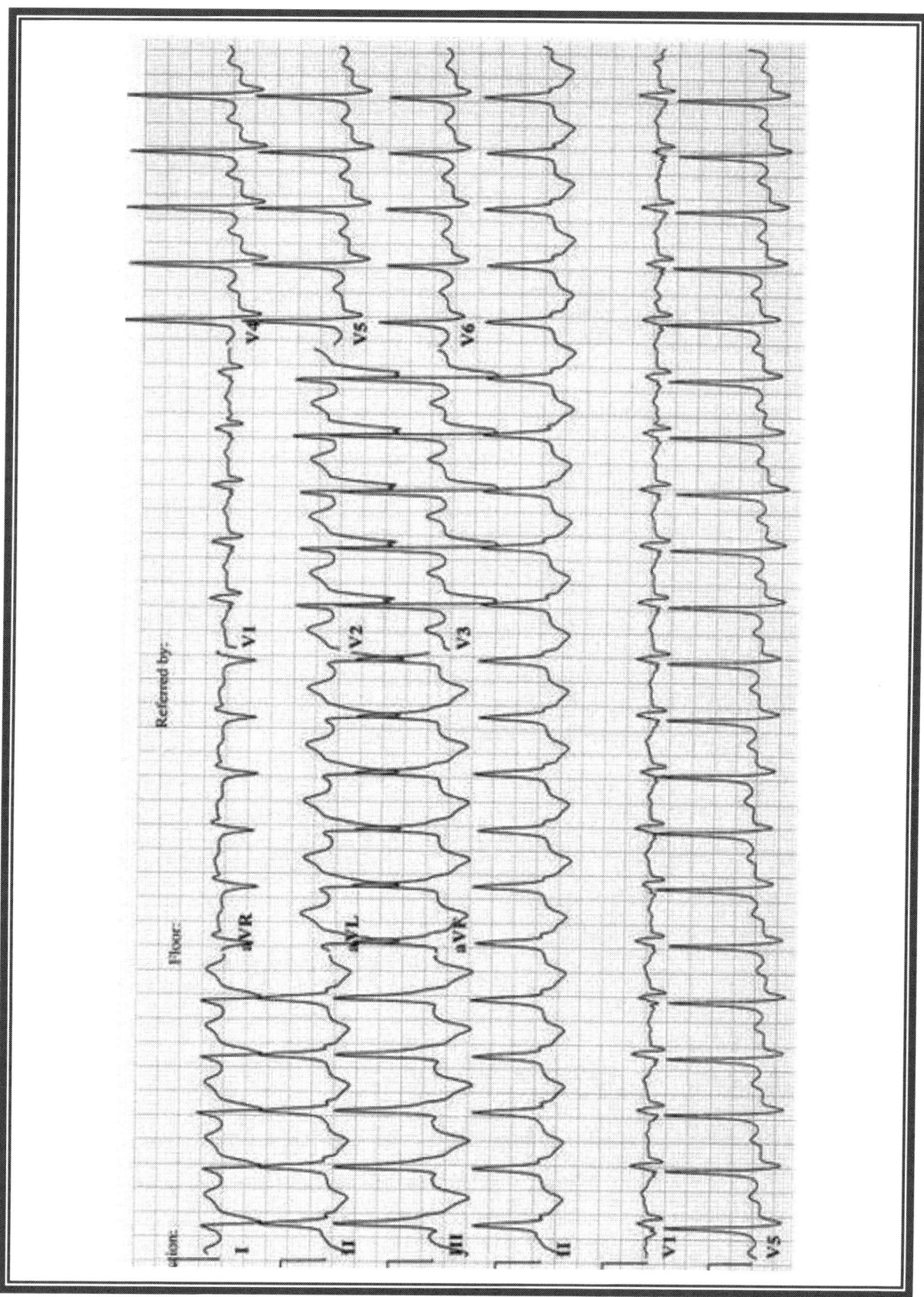

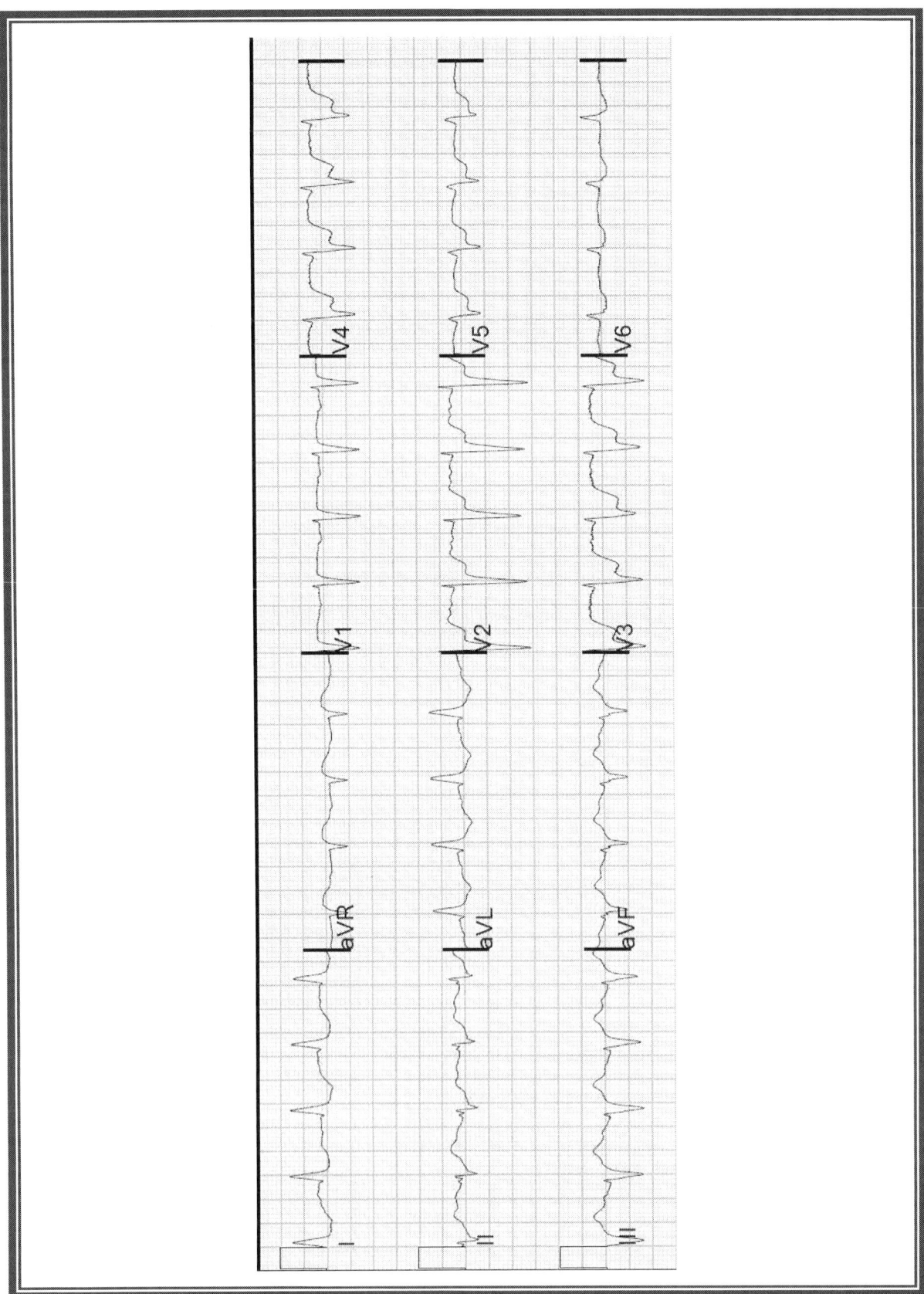

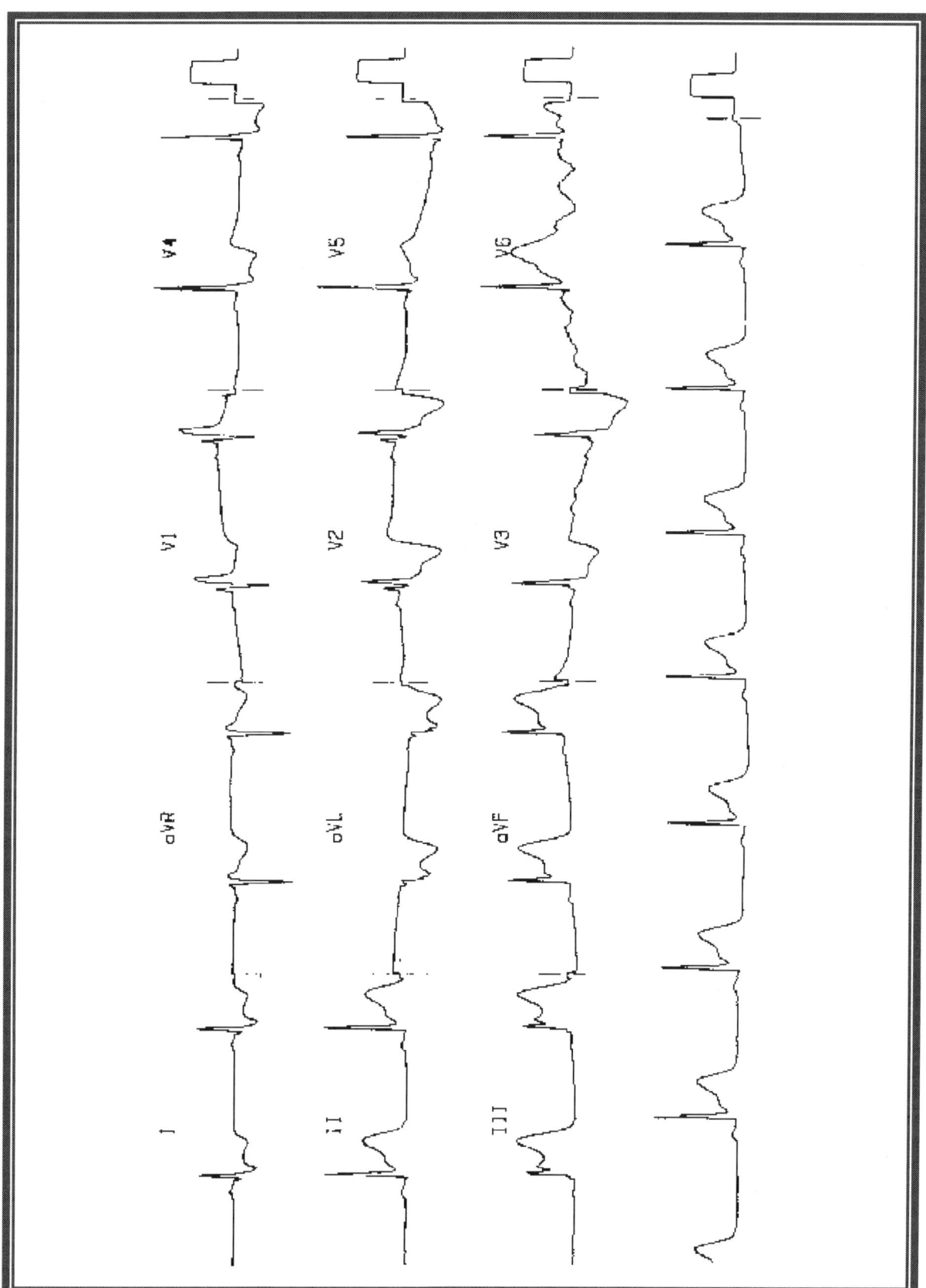

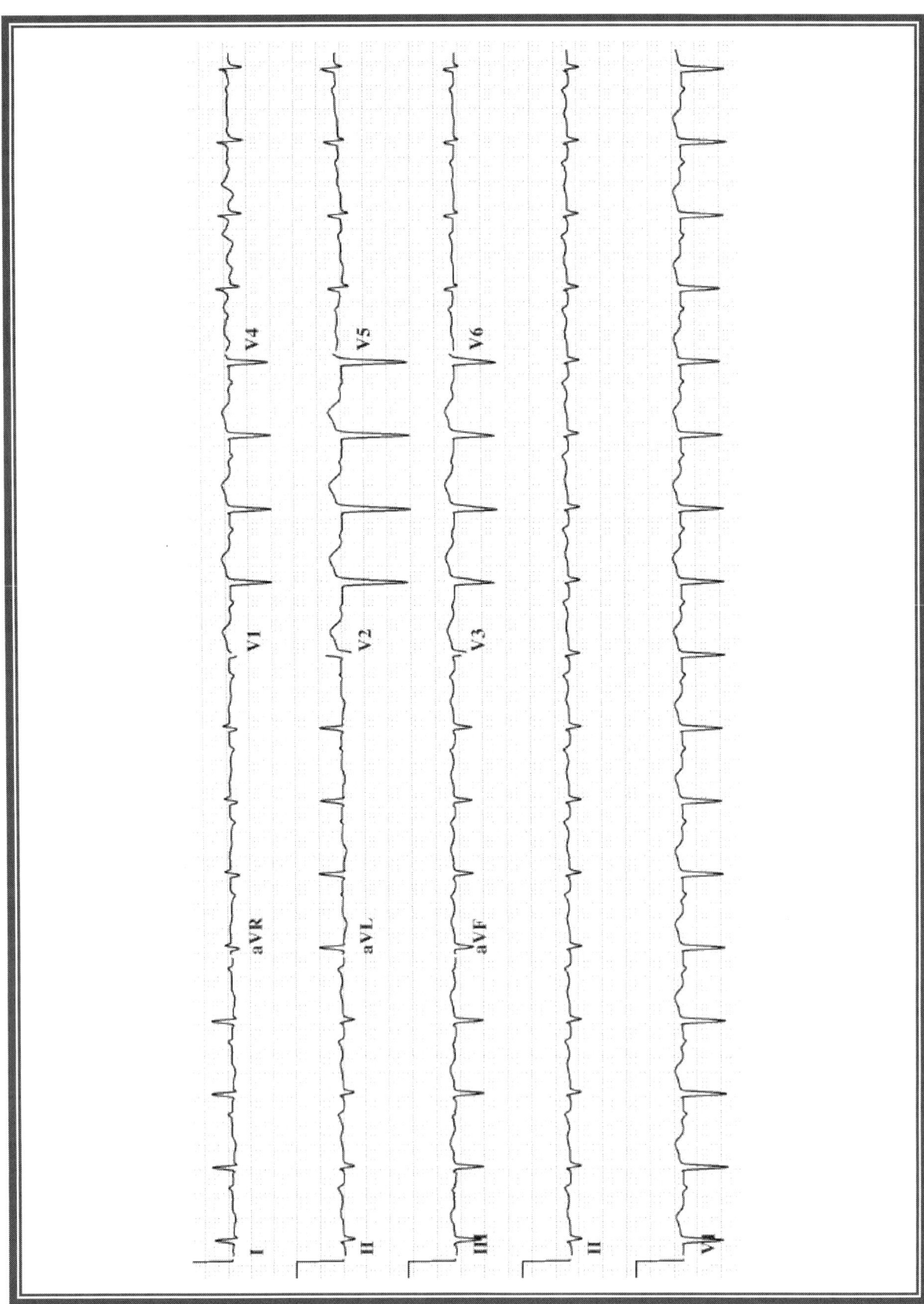

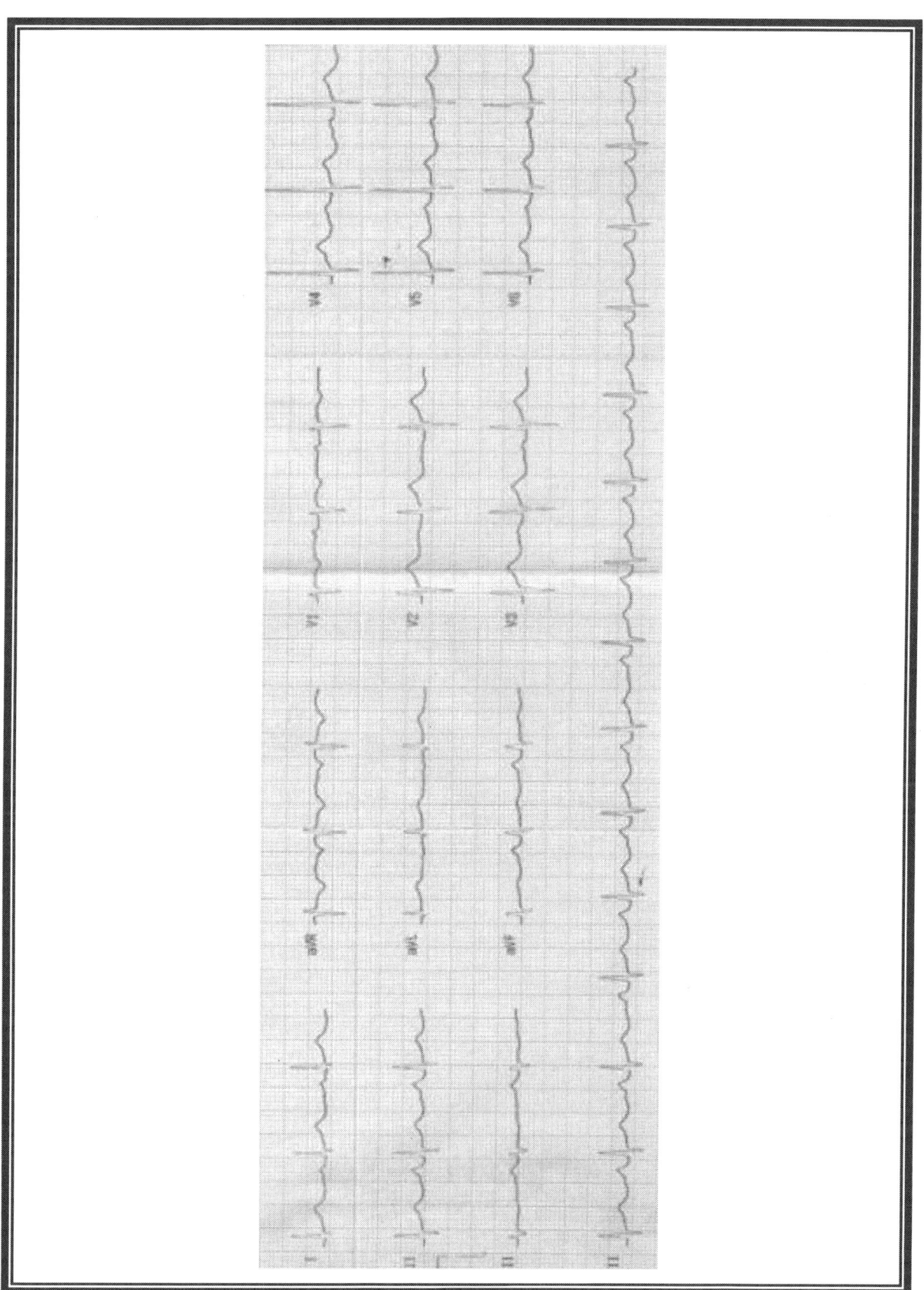

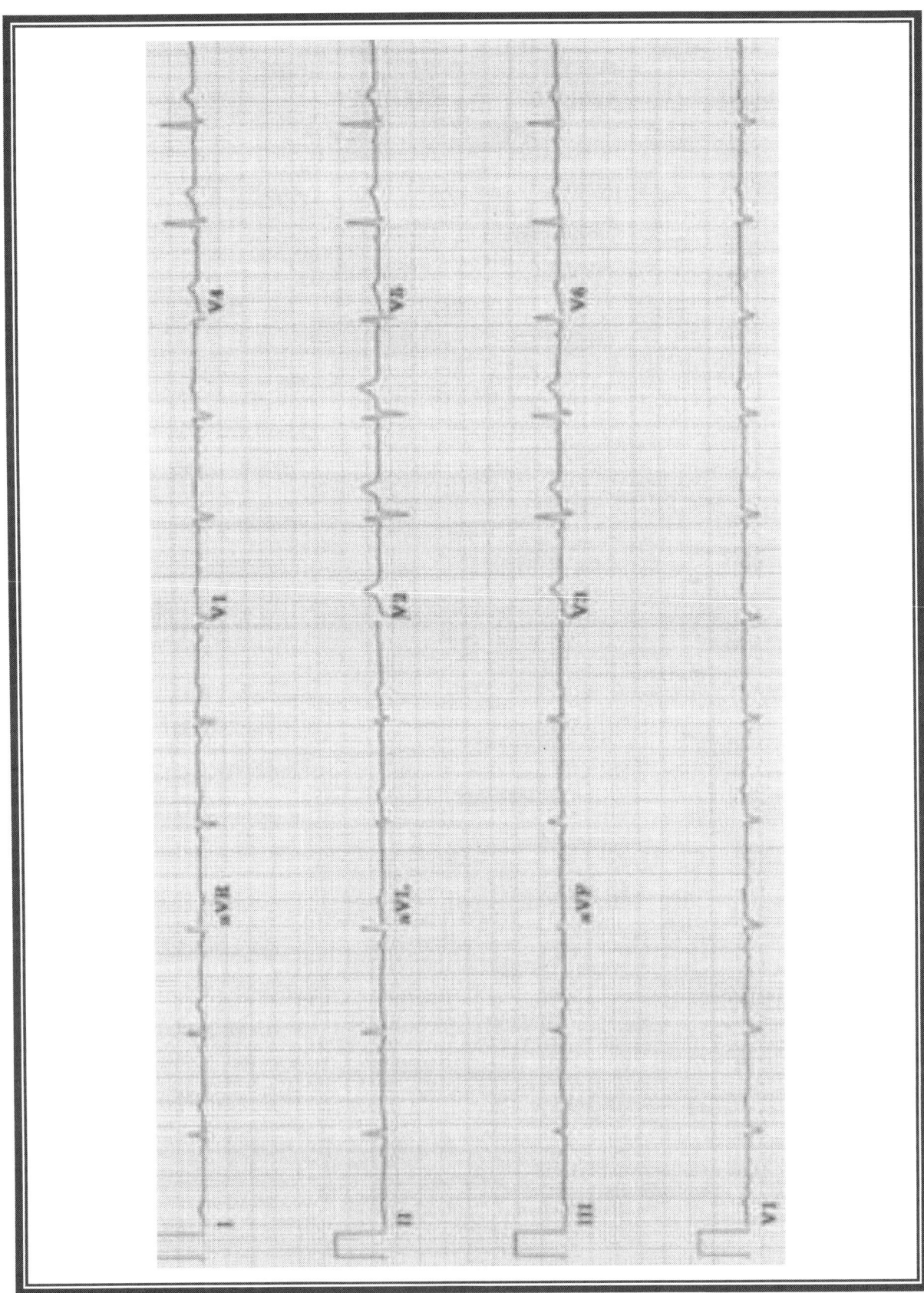

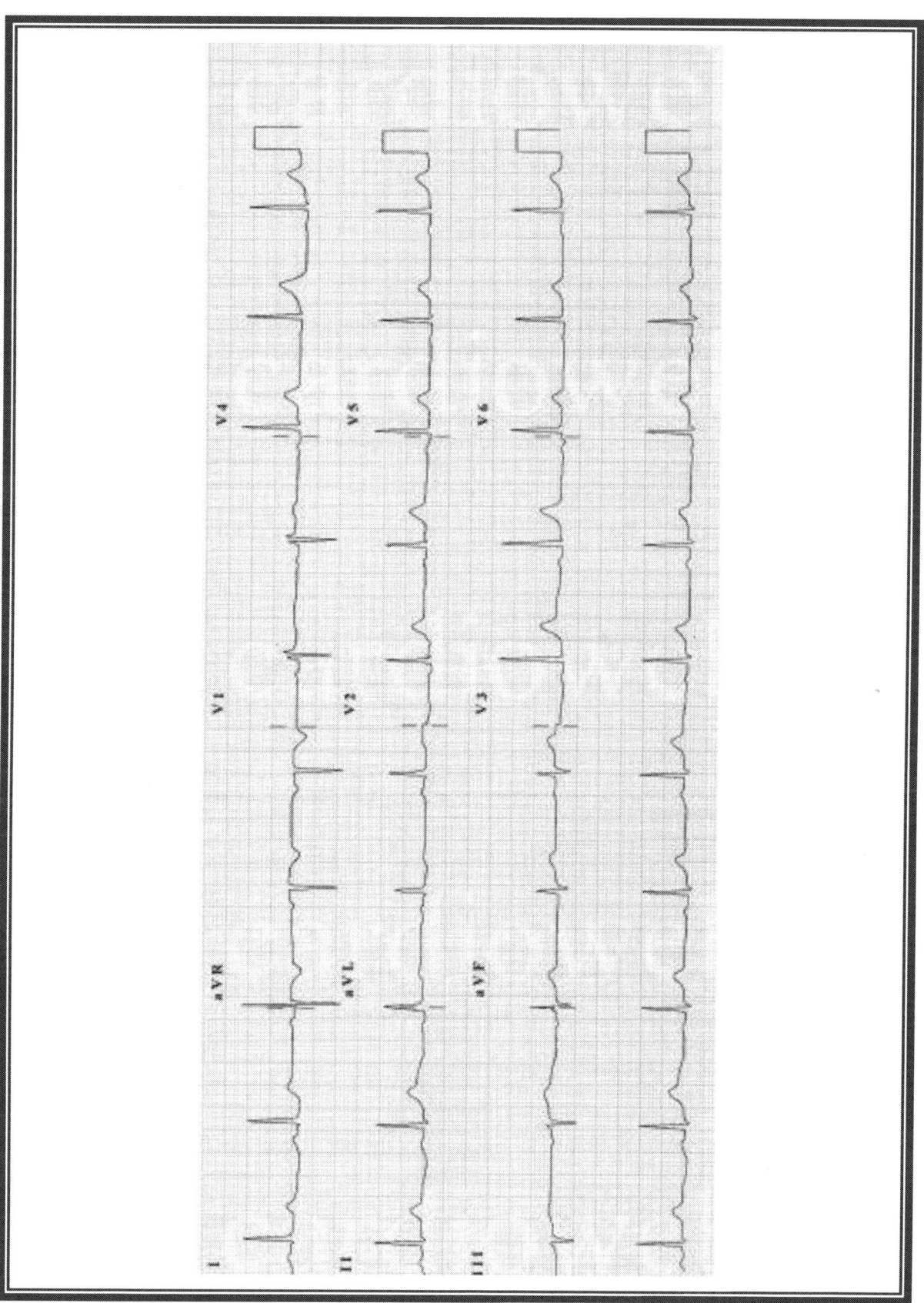

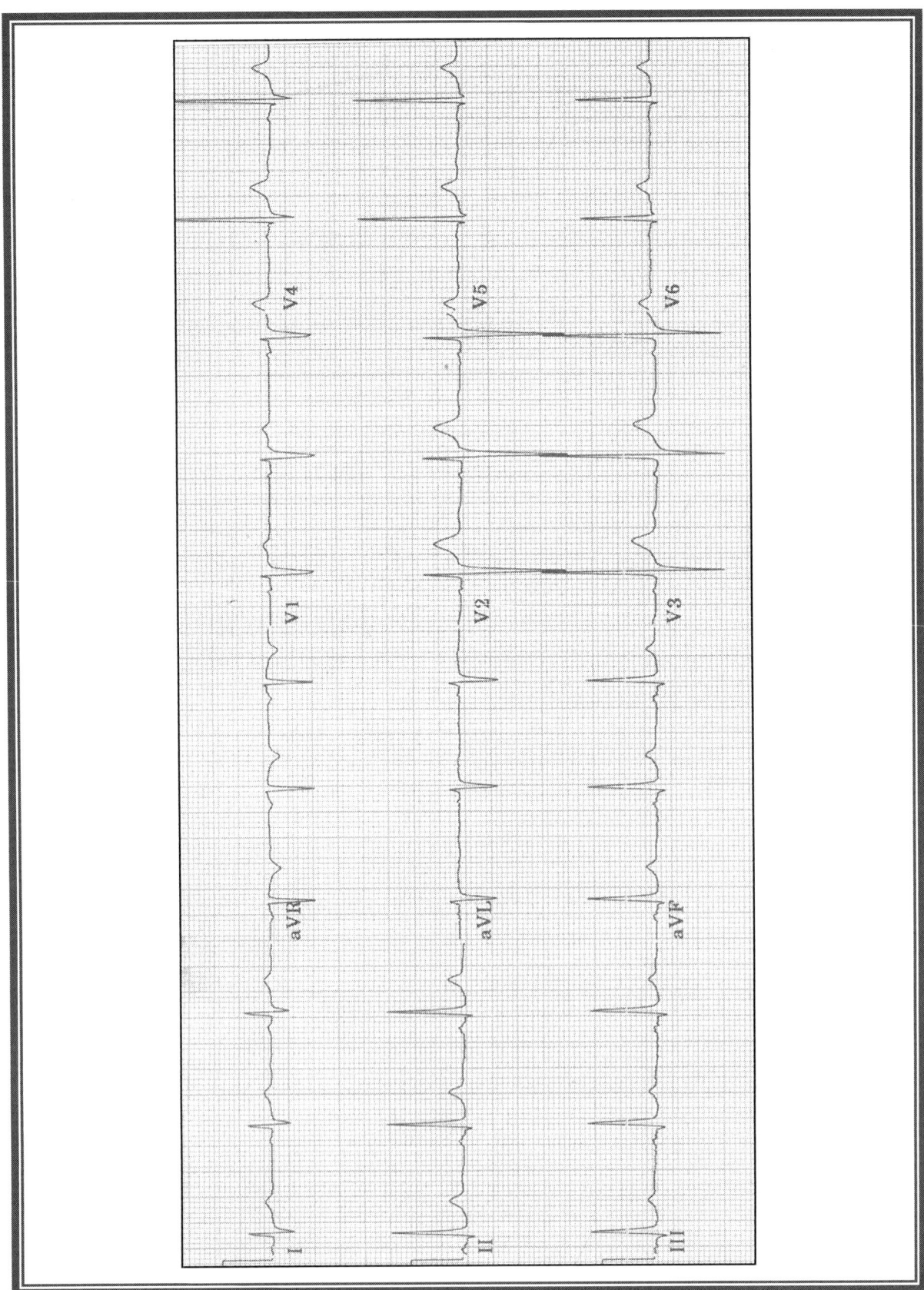

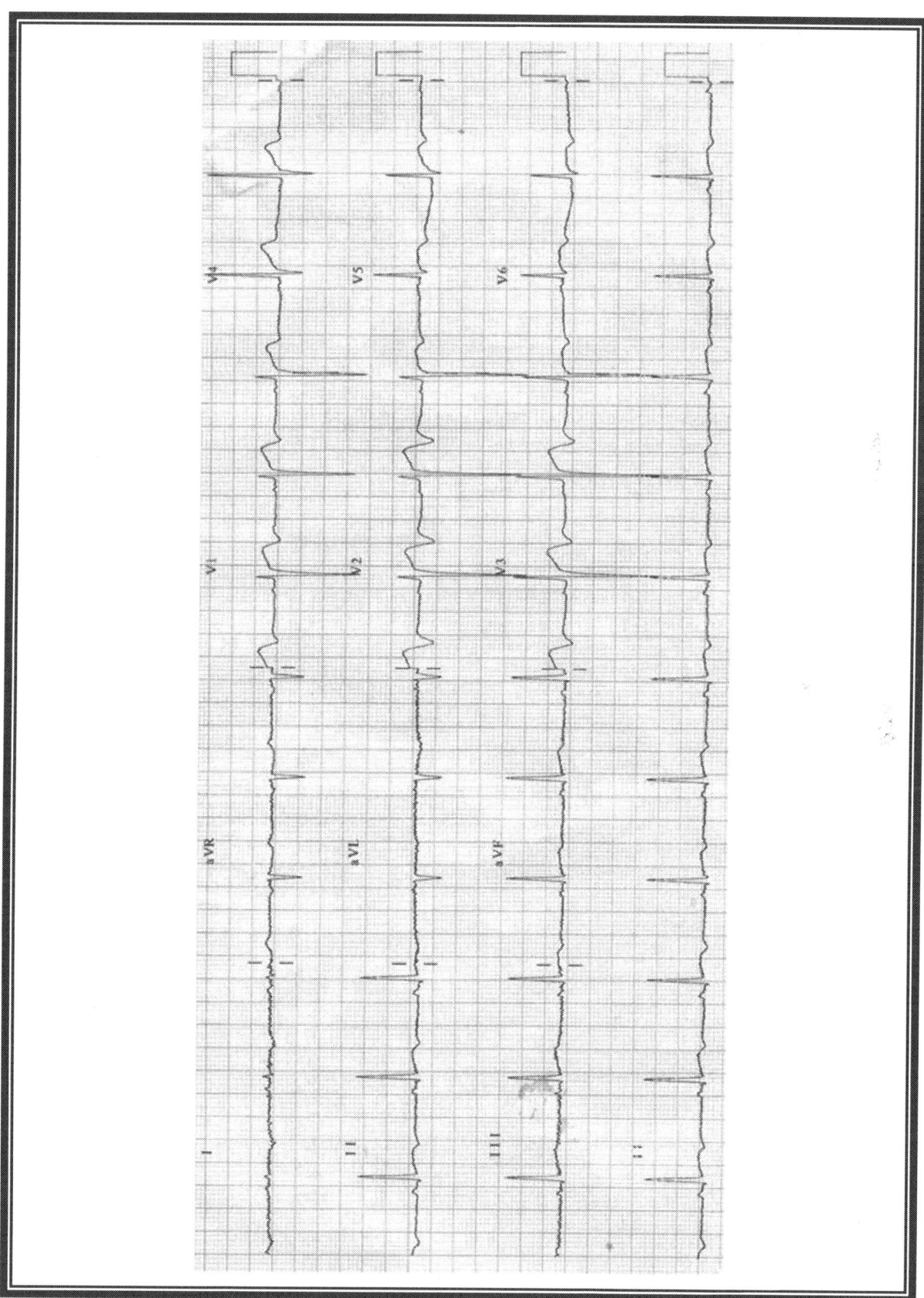

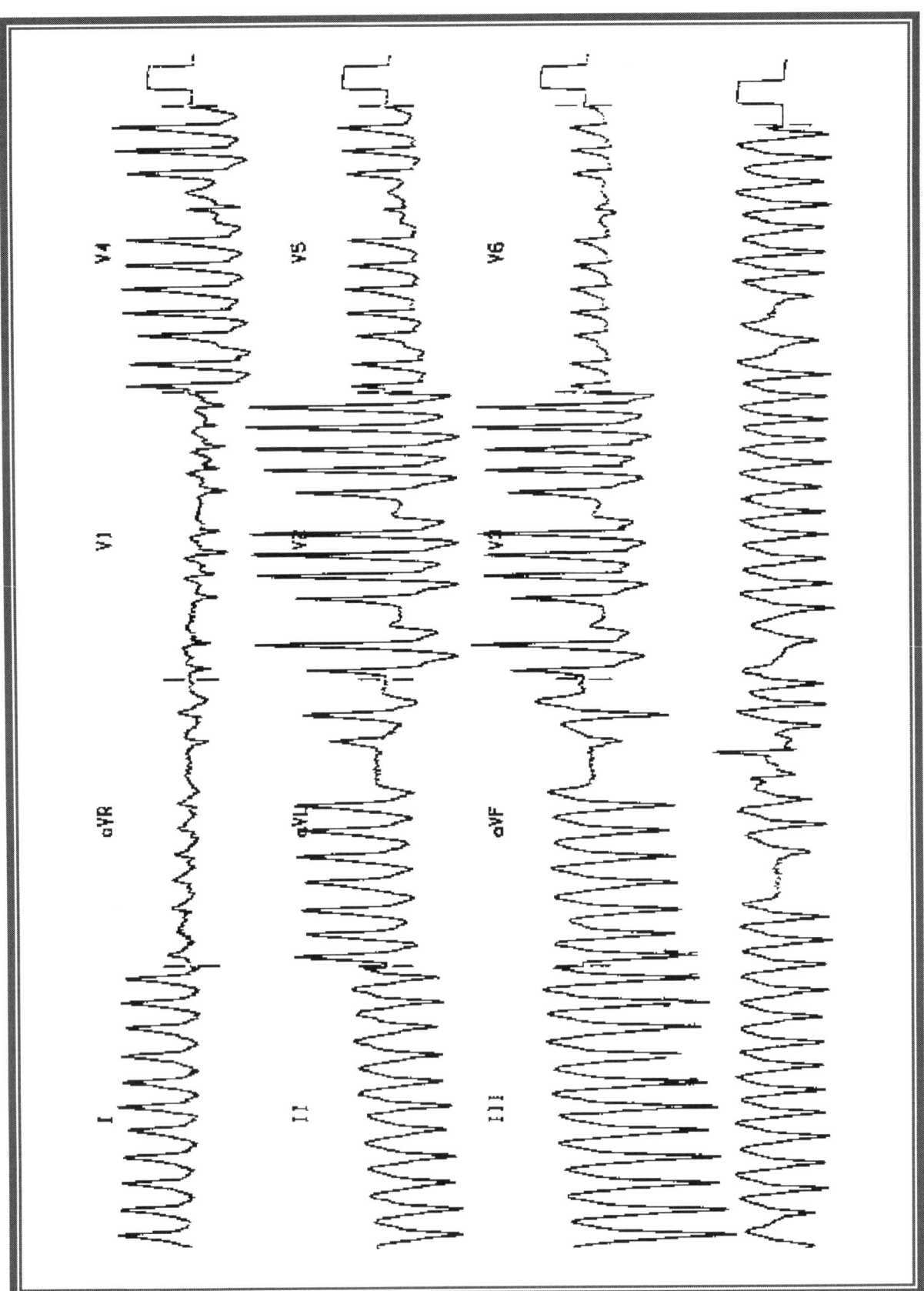

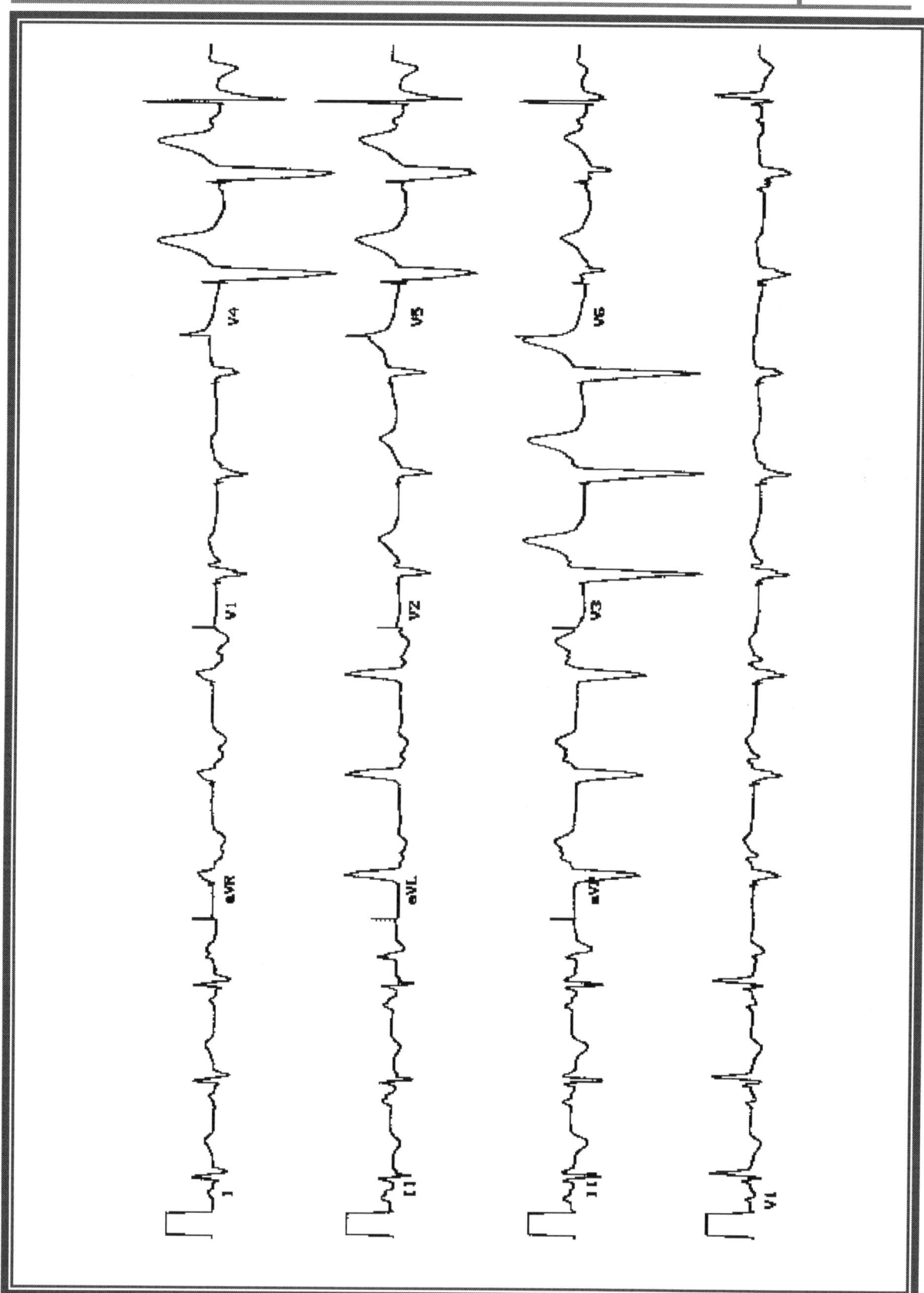

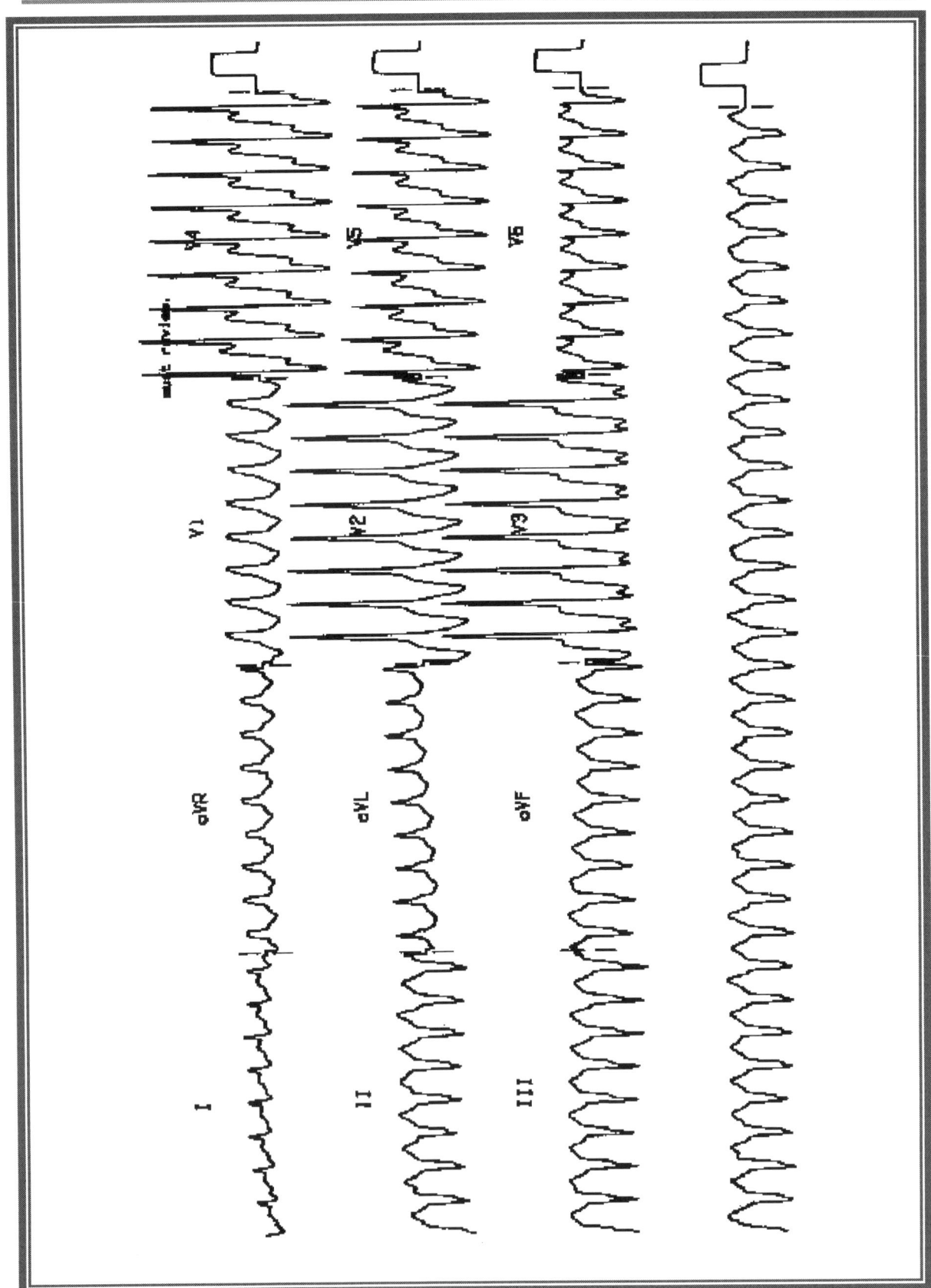

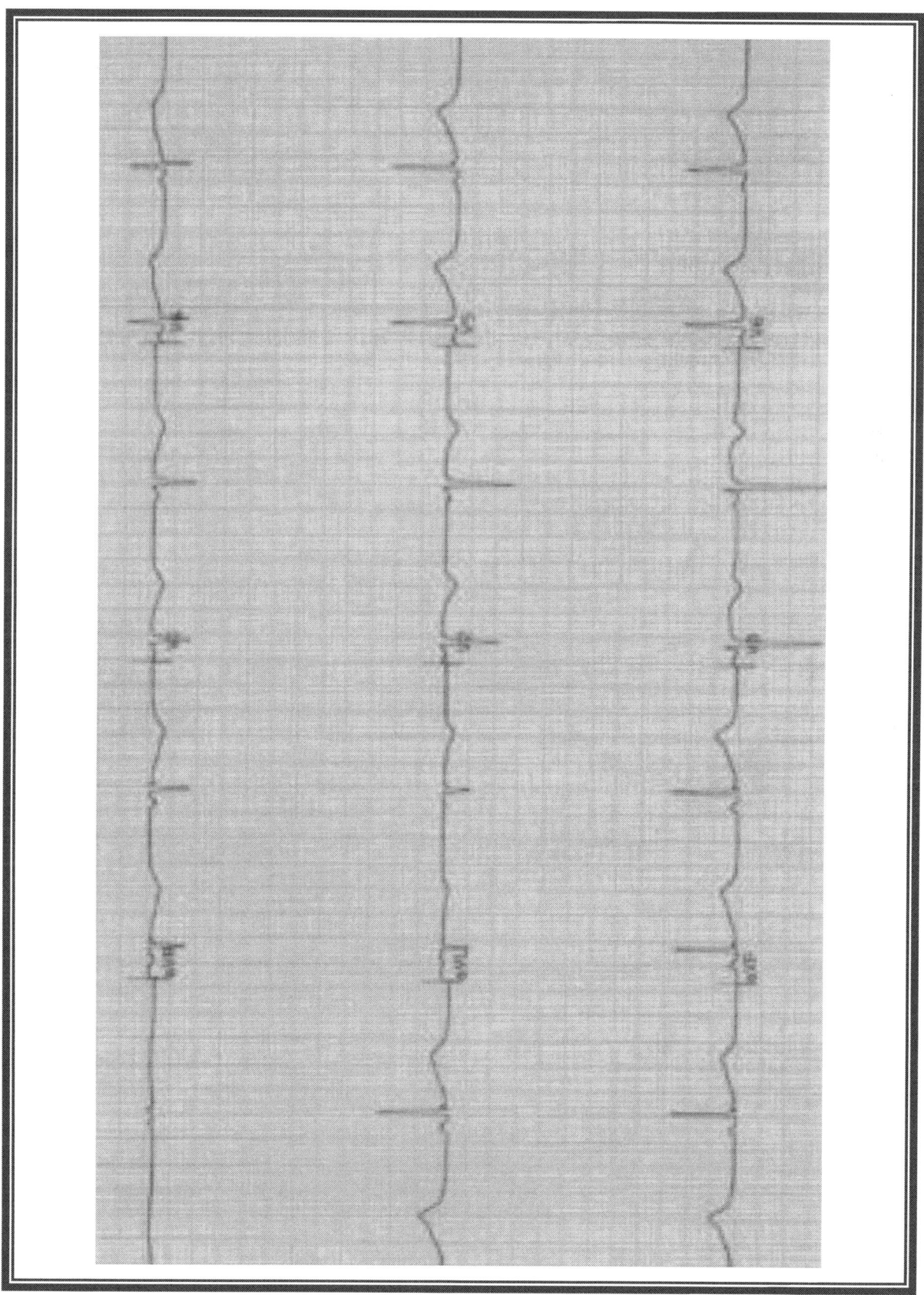

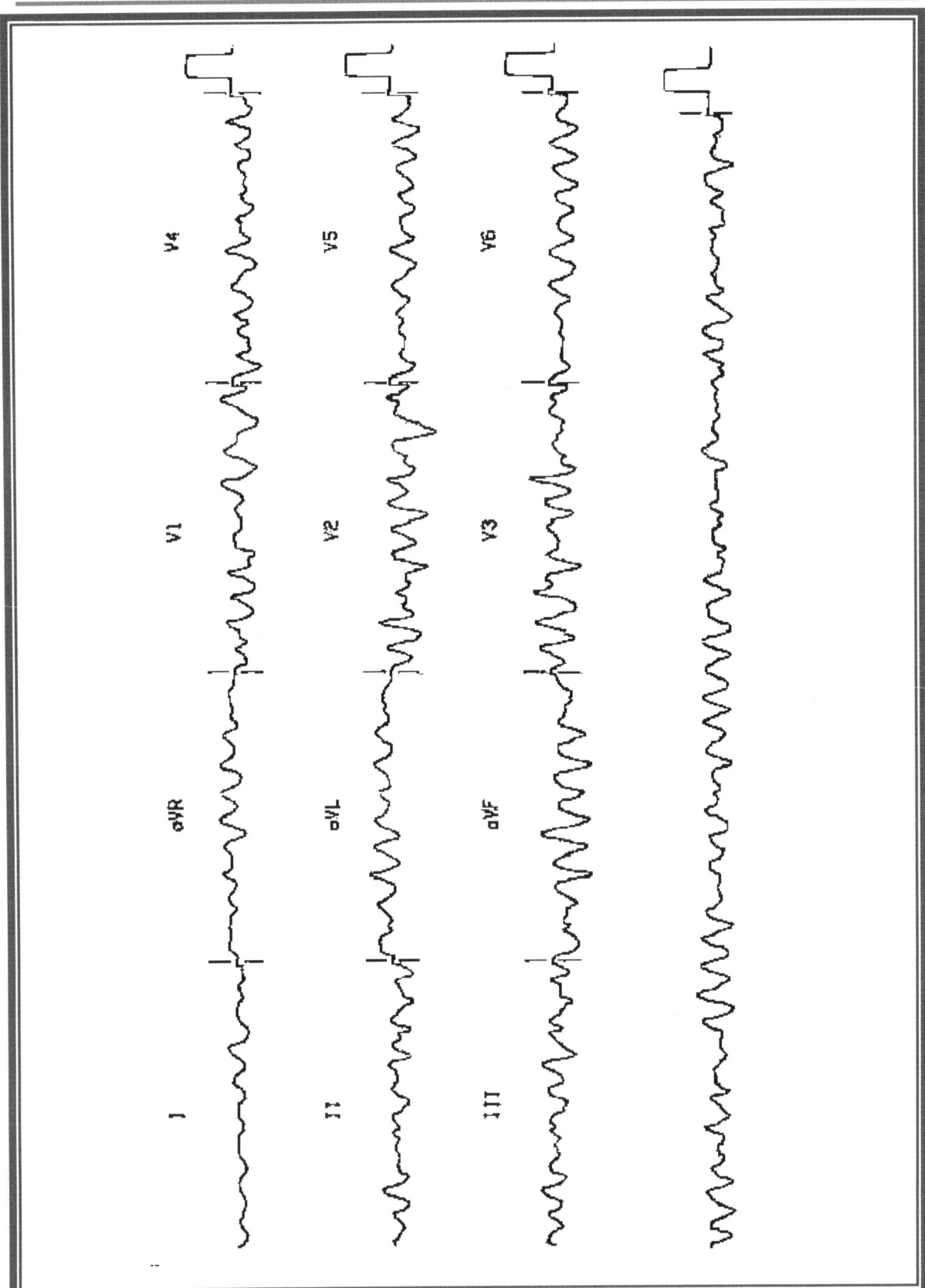

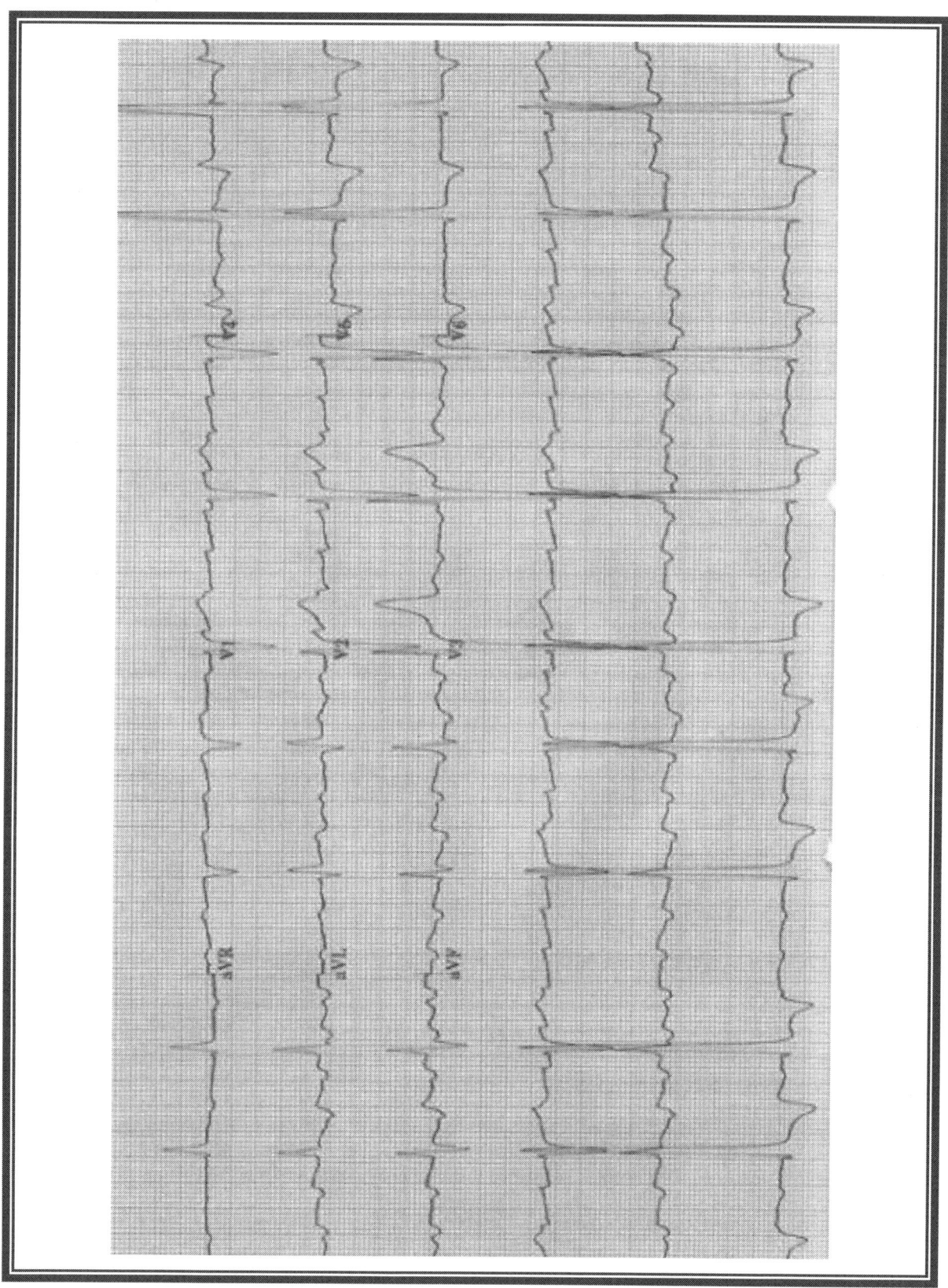

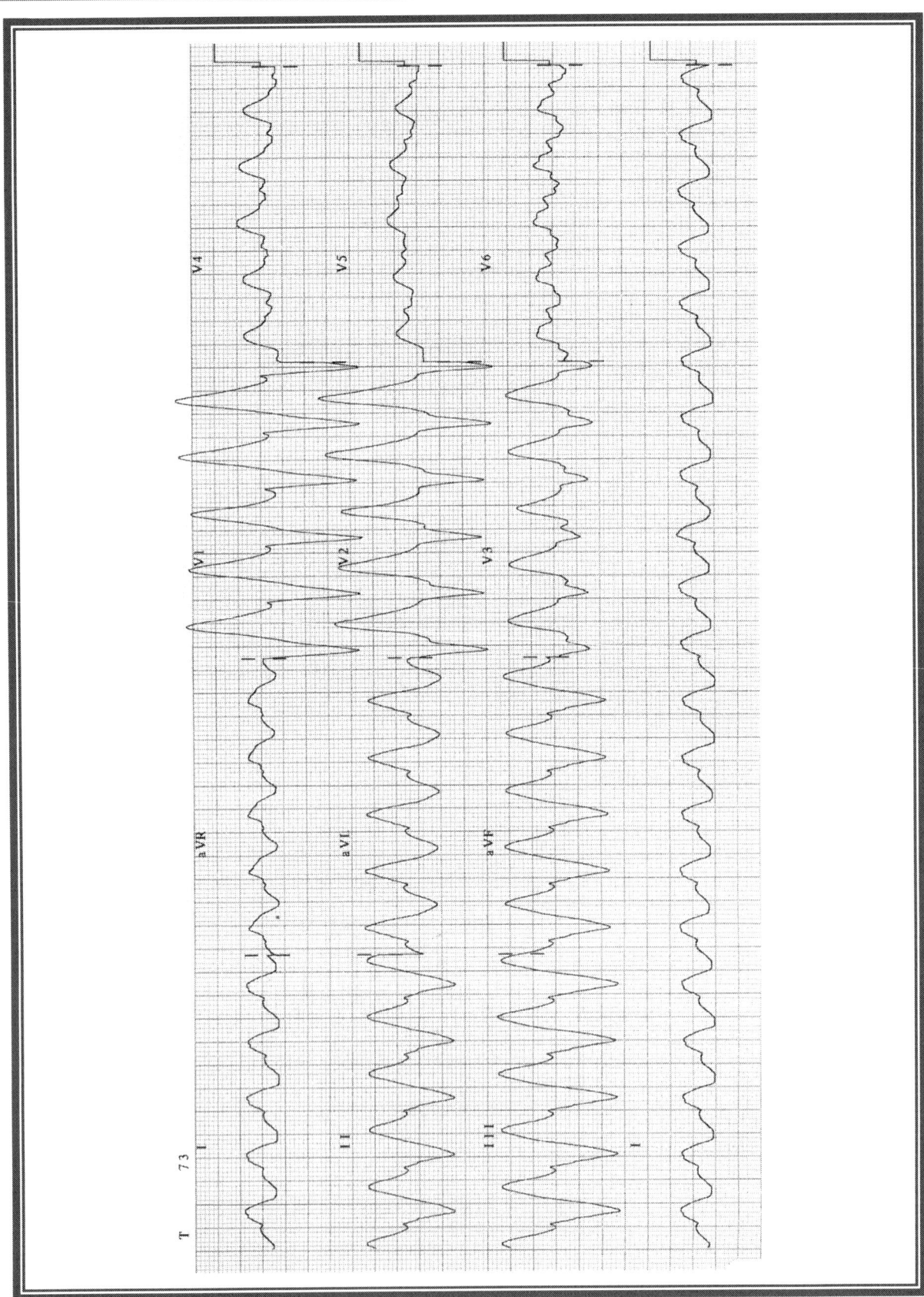

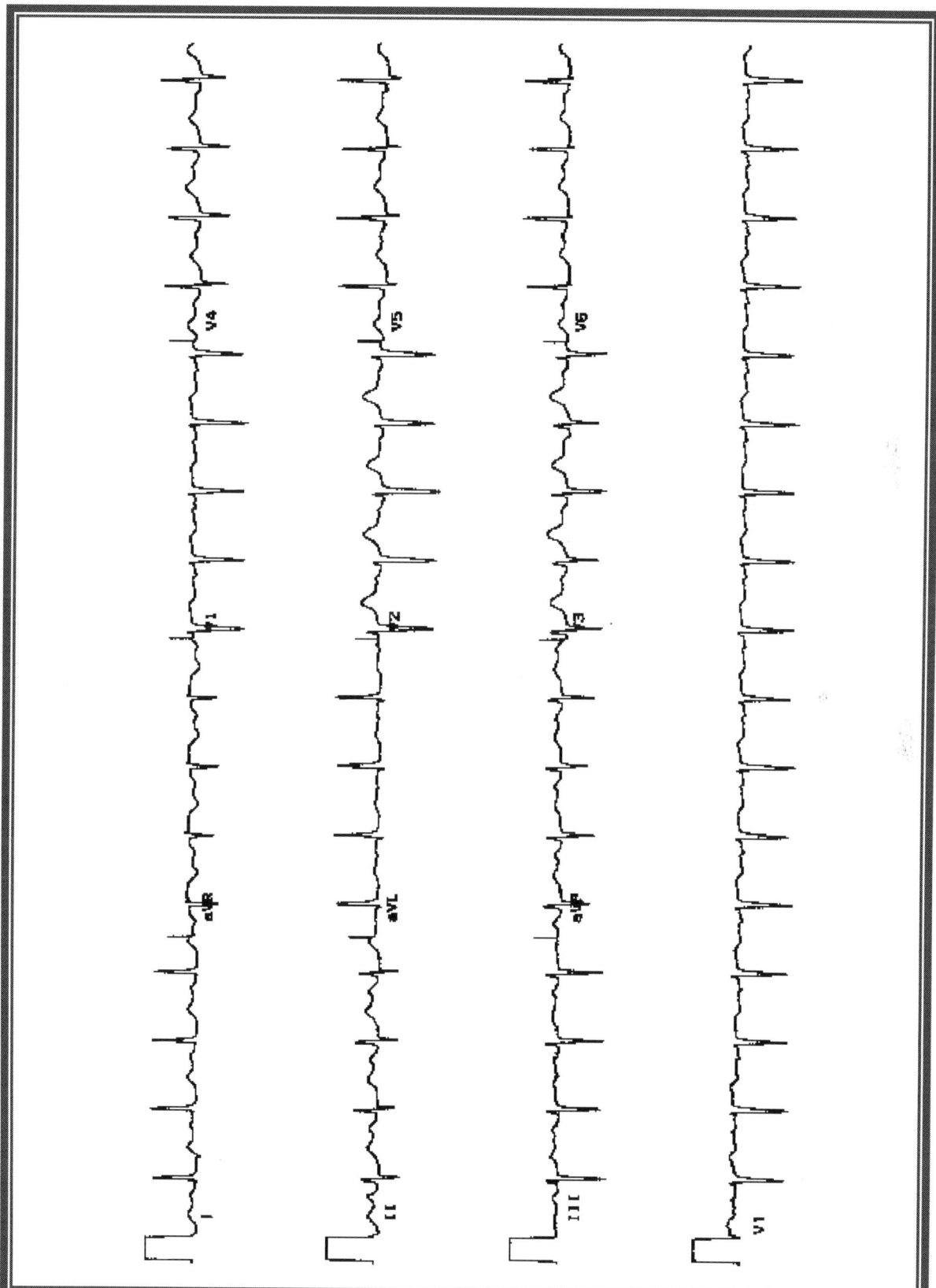

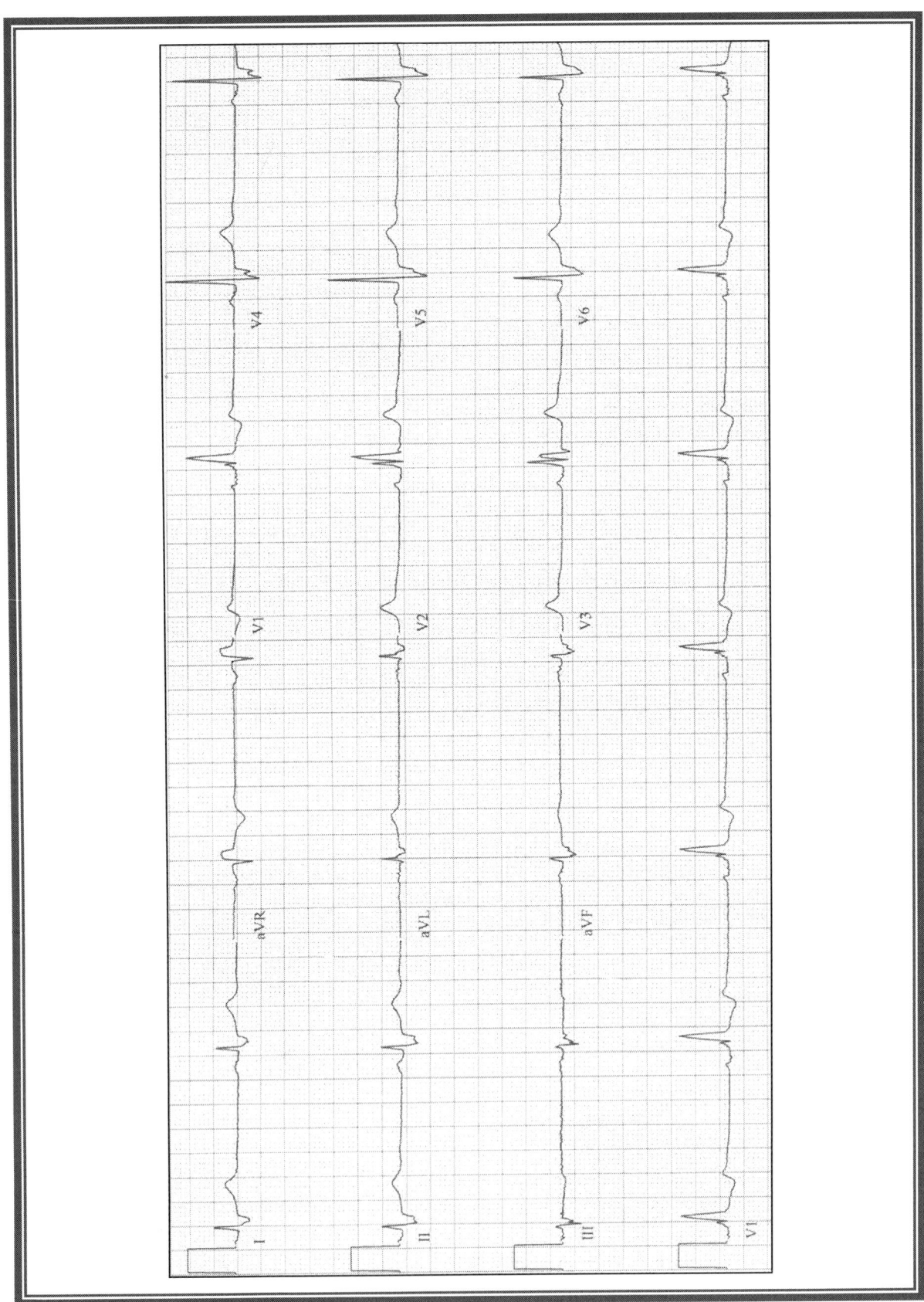

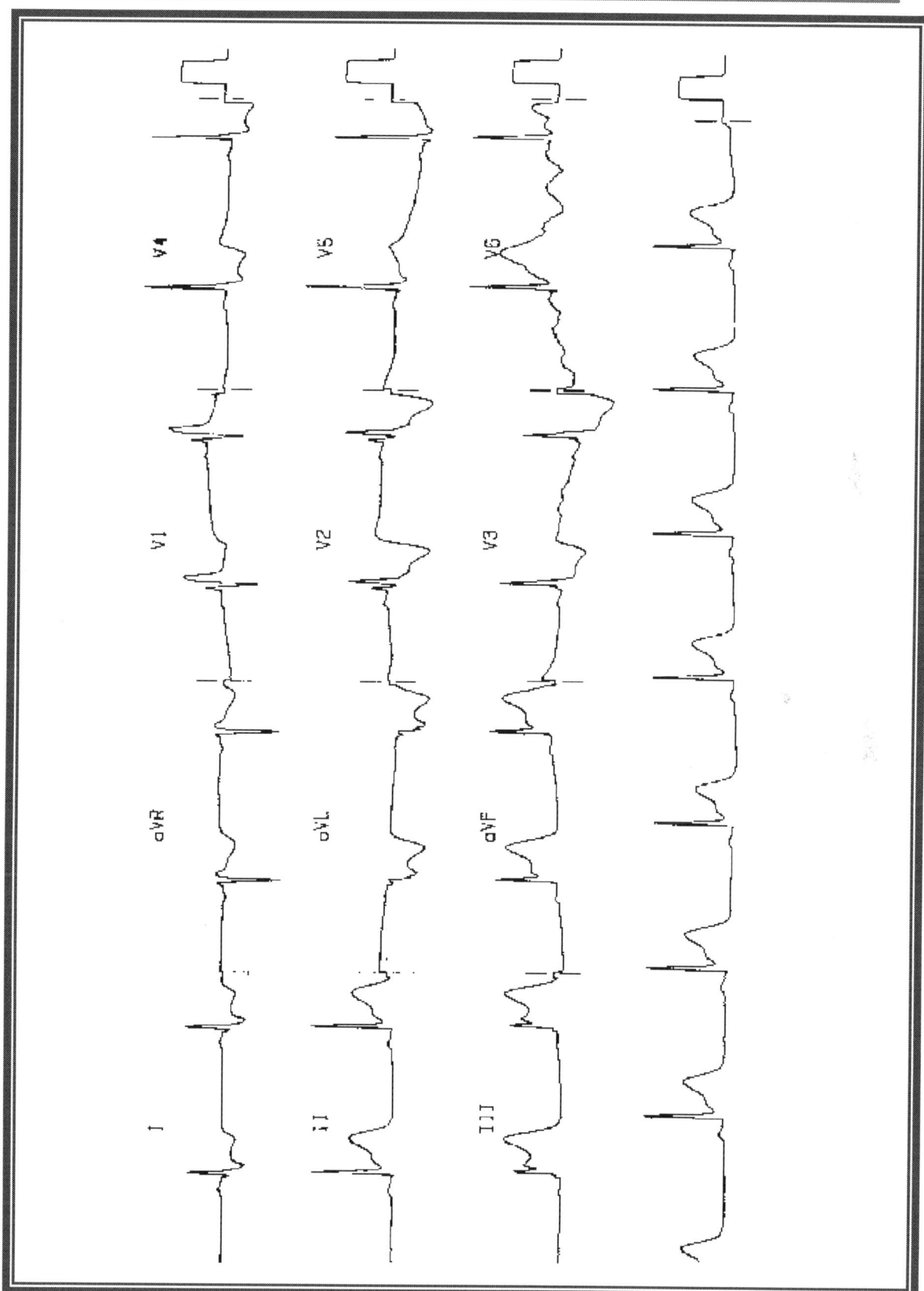

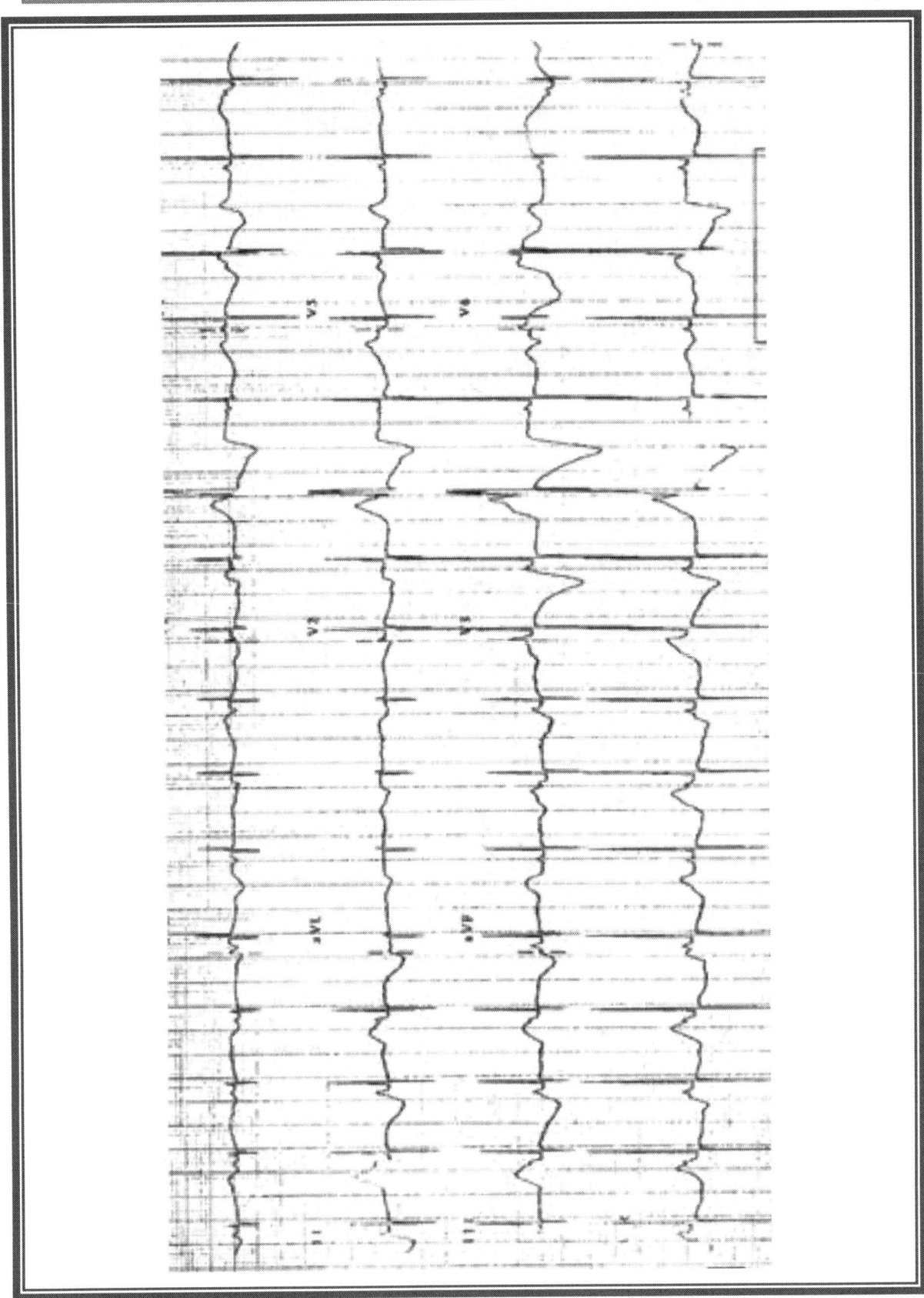

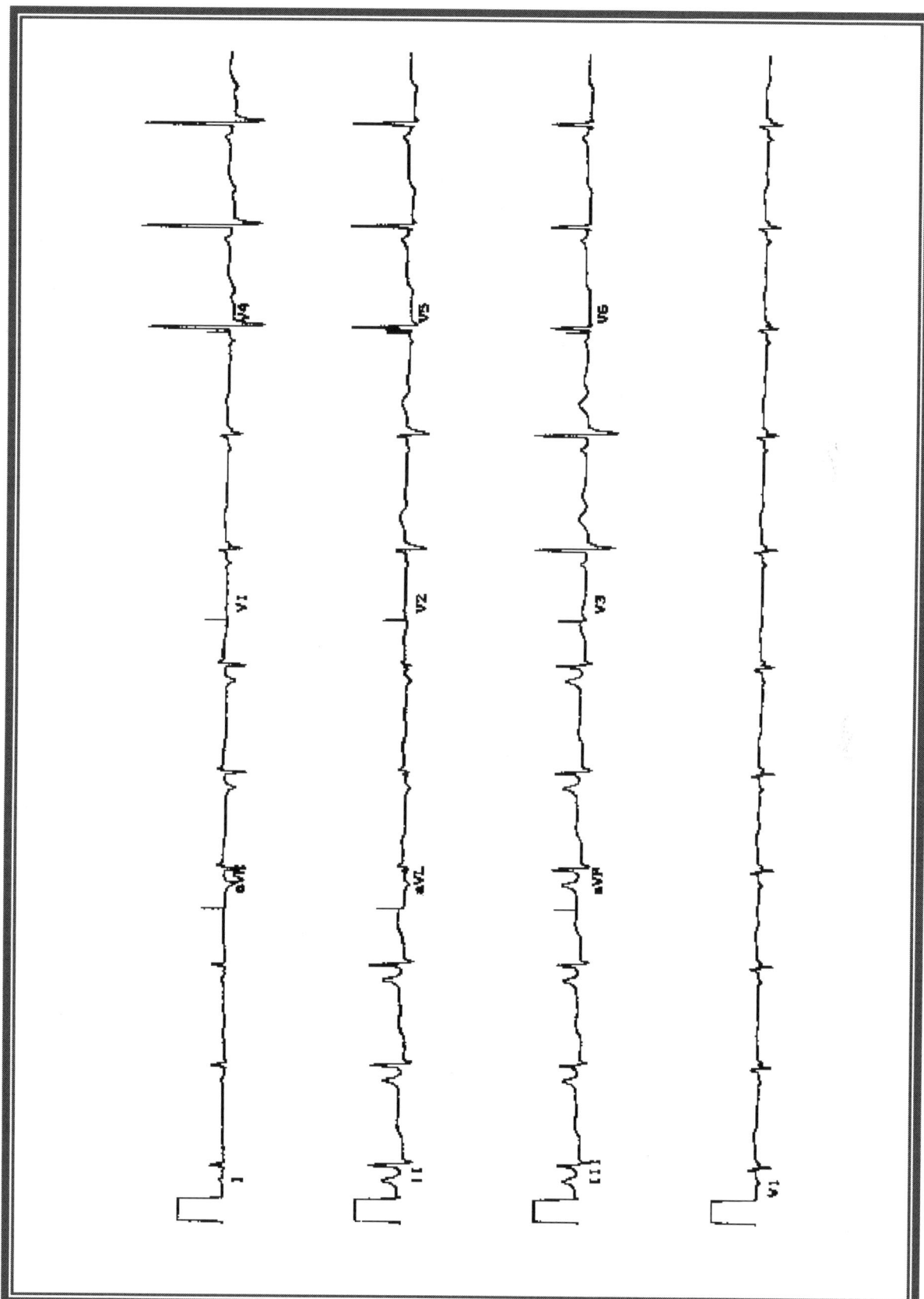

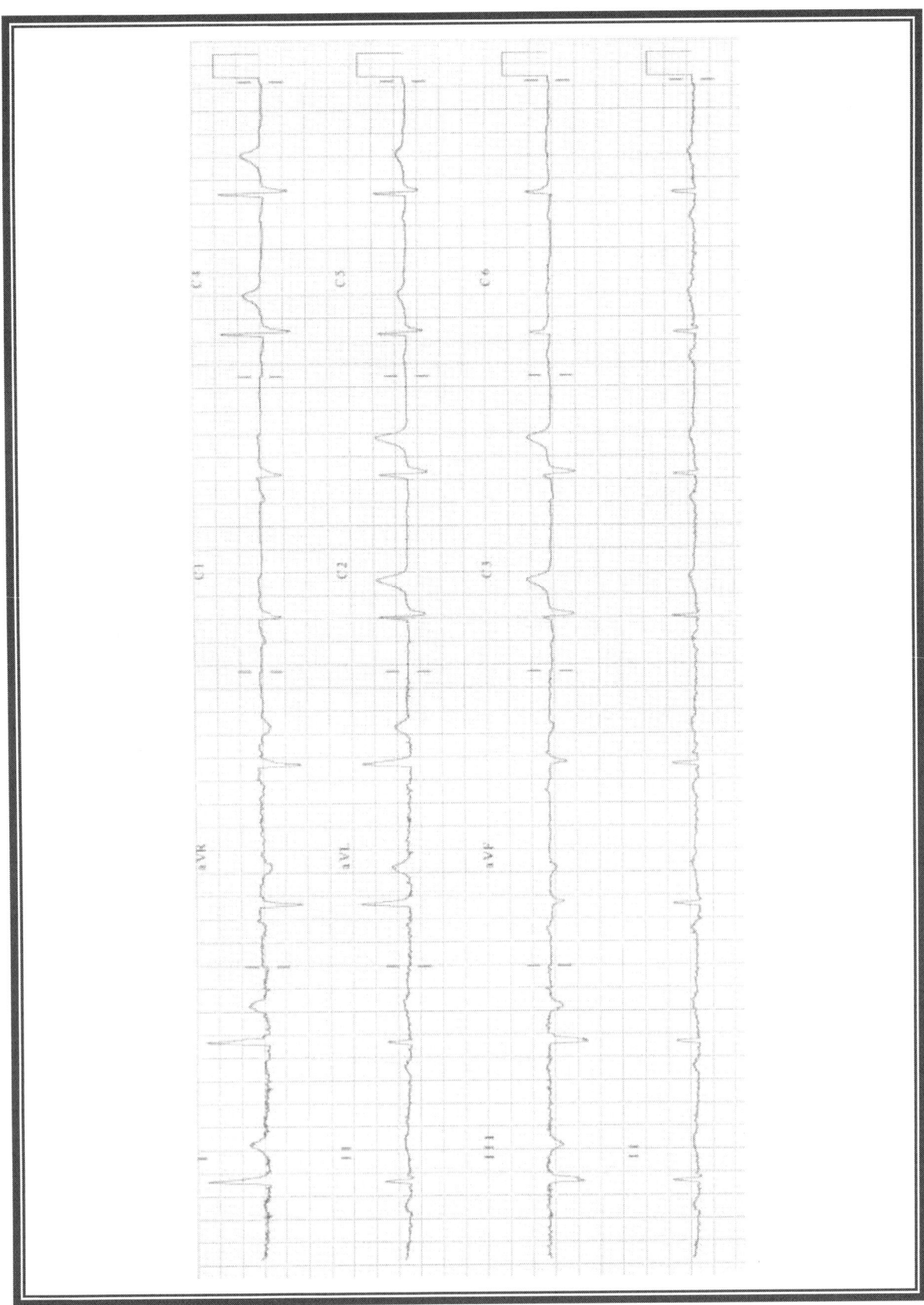

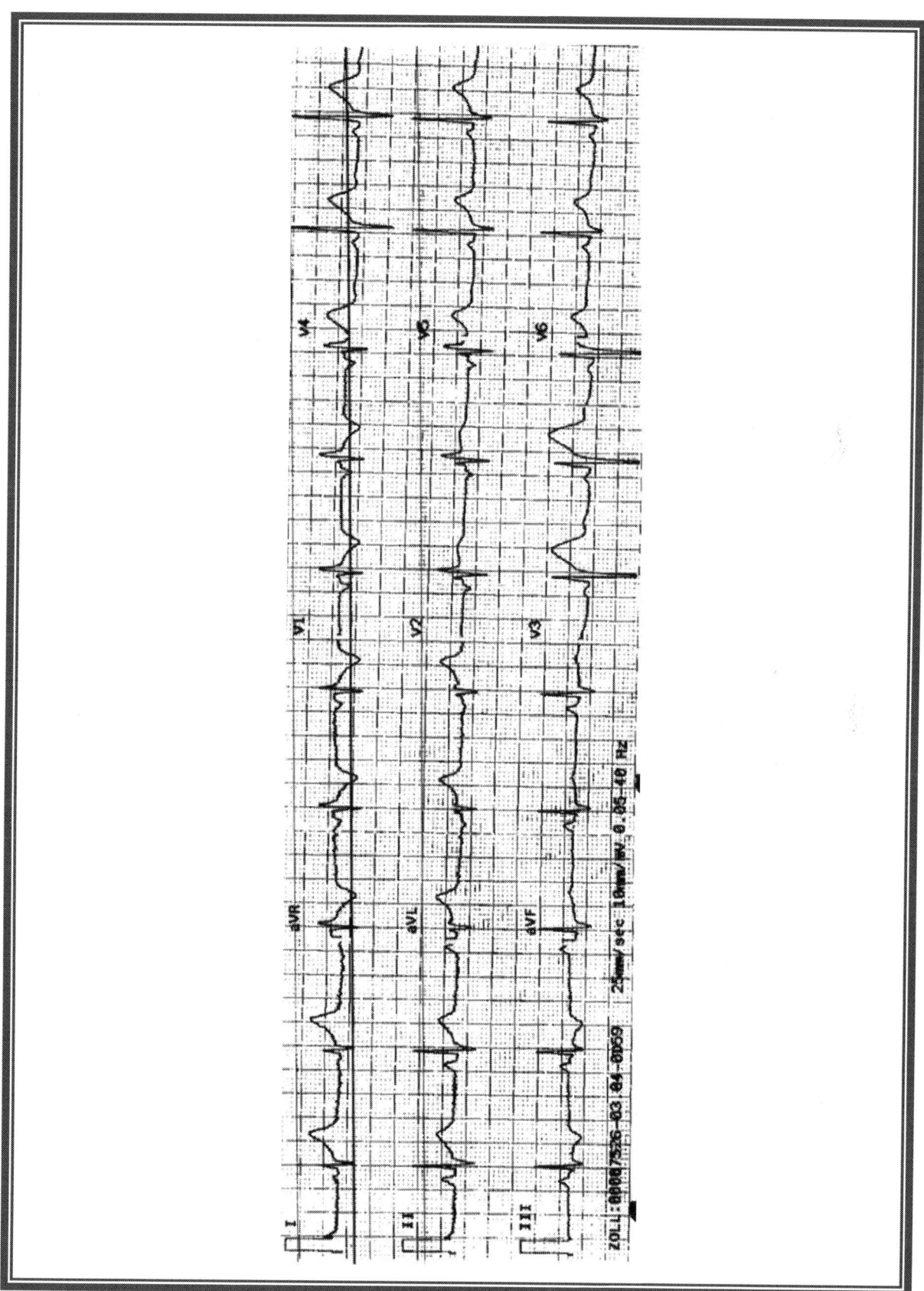

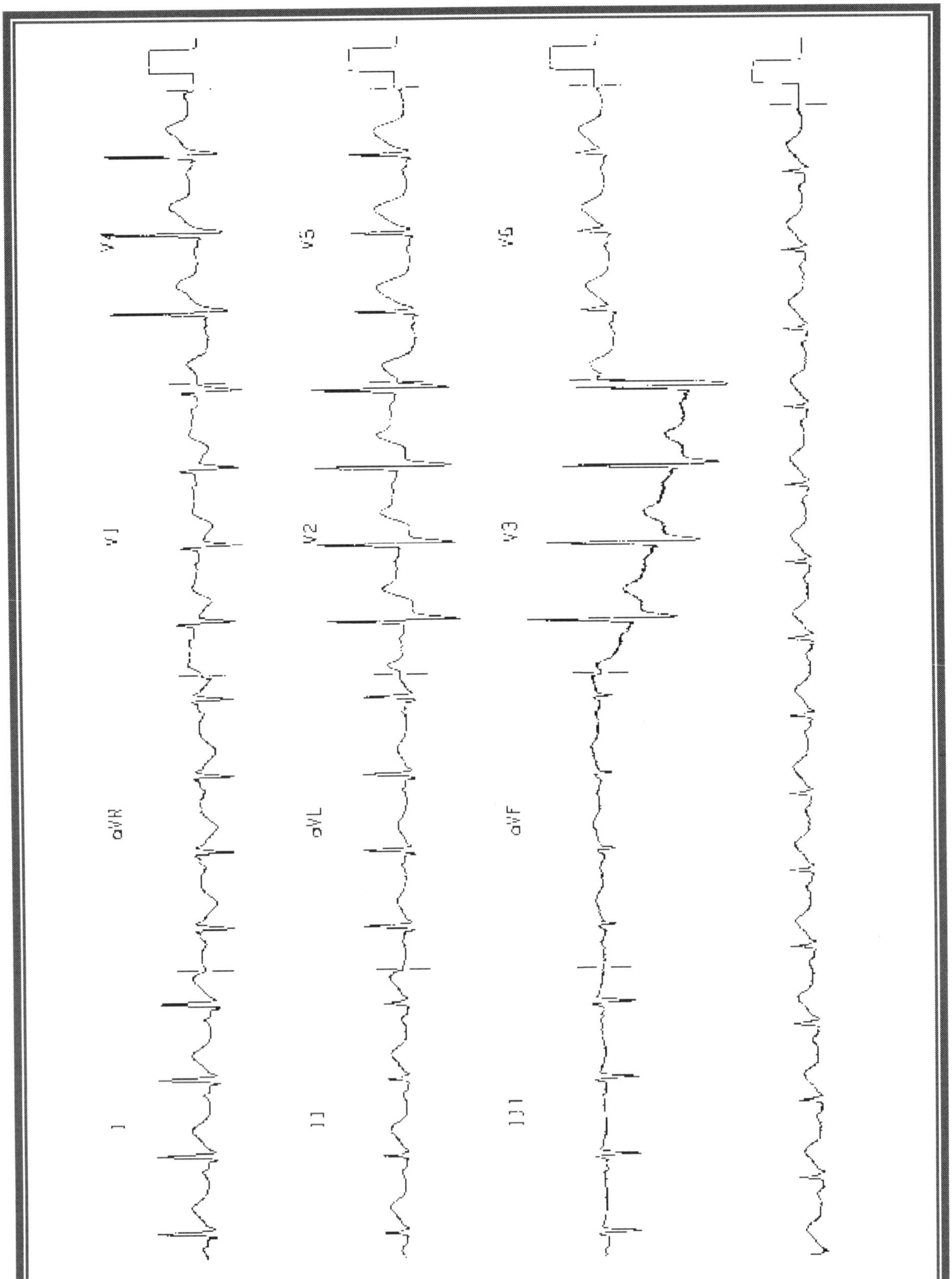
I
aVR
V1
V4
II
aVL
V2
V5
III
aVF
V3

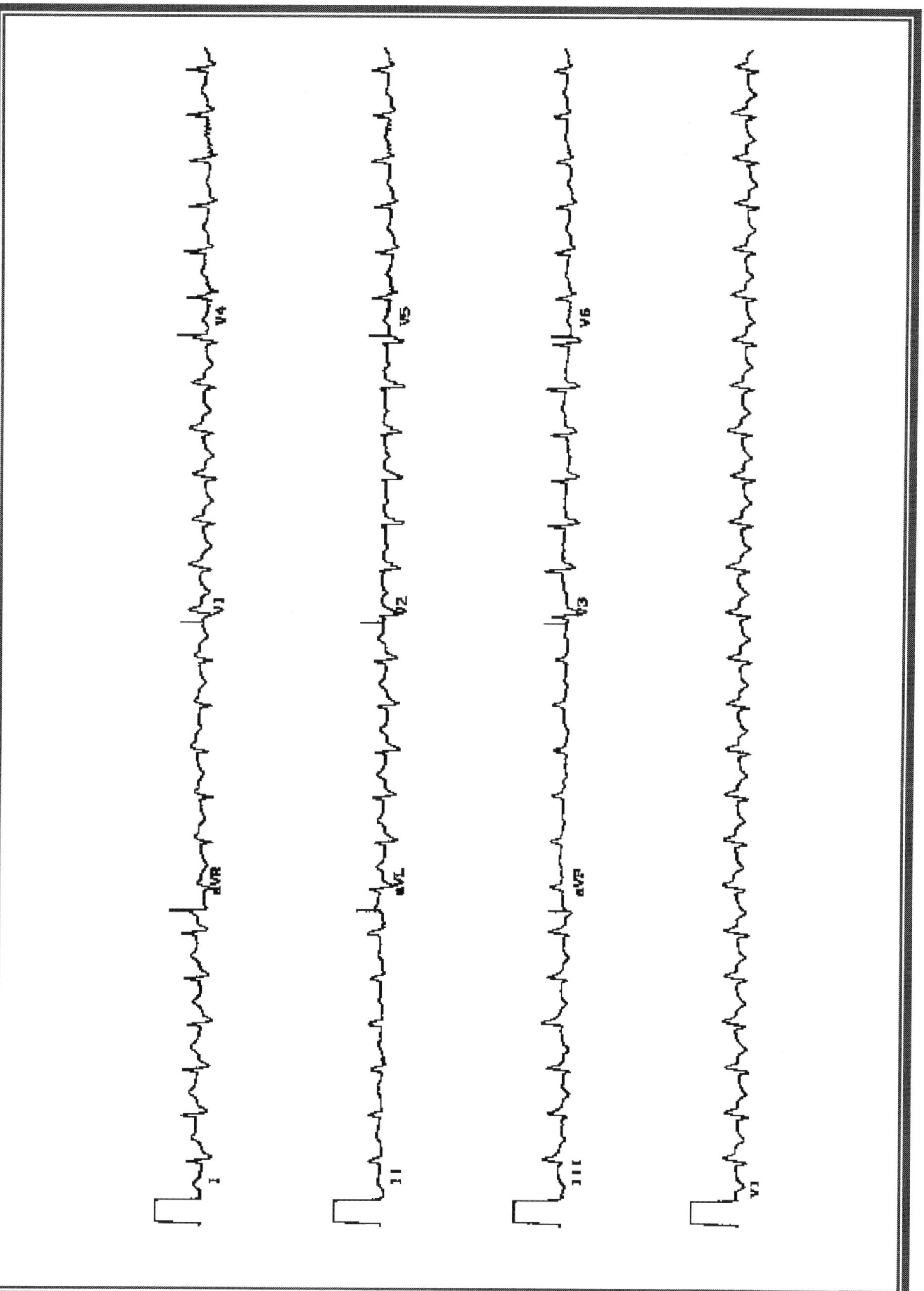
I
aVR
V1
V4
II
aVL
V2
V5
III
aVF
V3
V6
V1

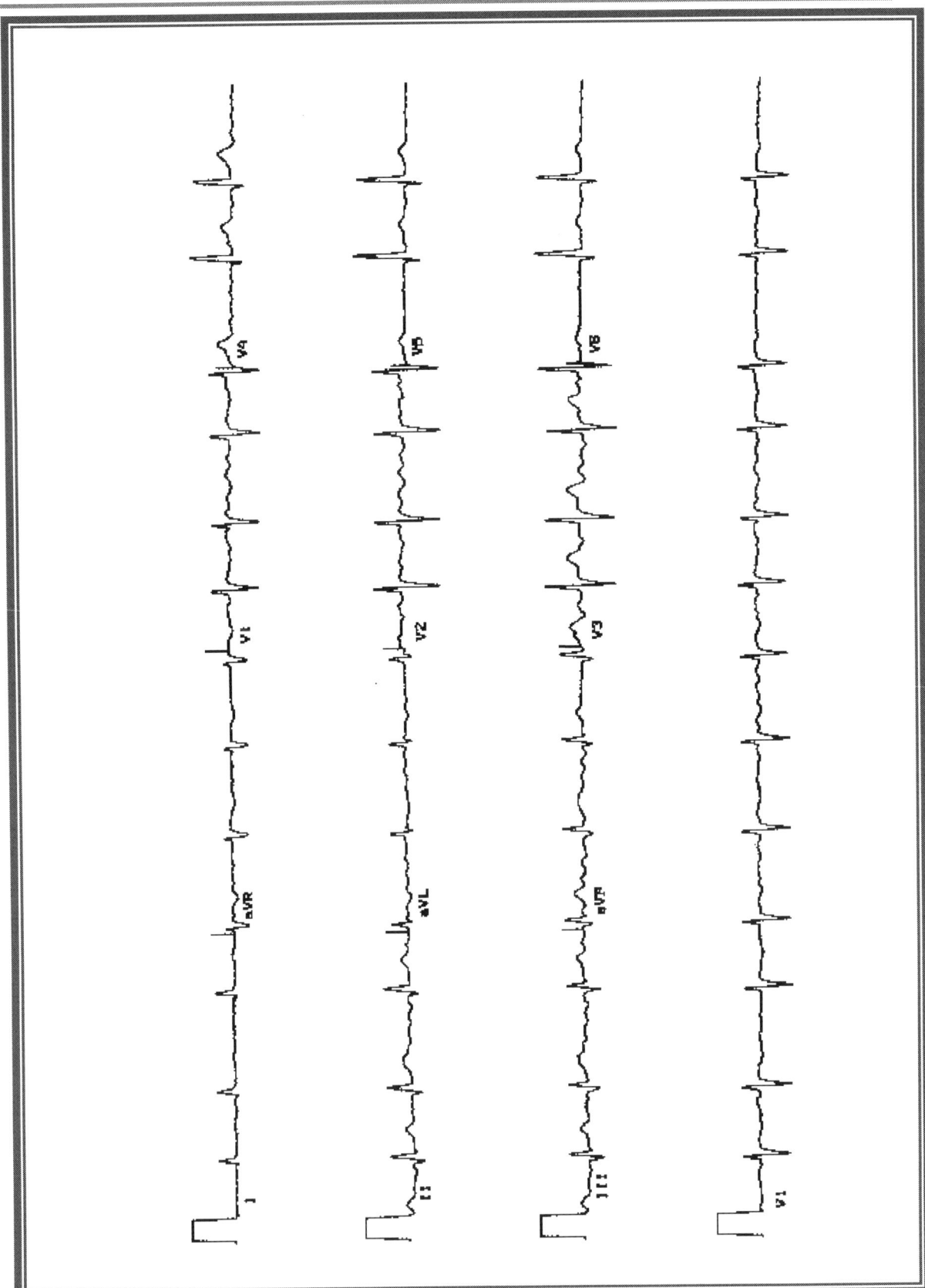

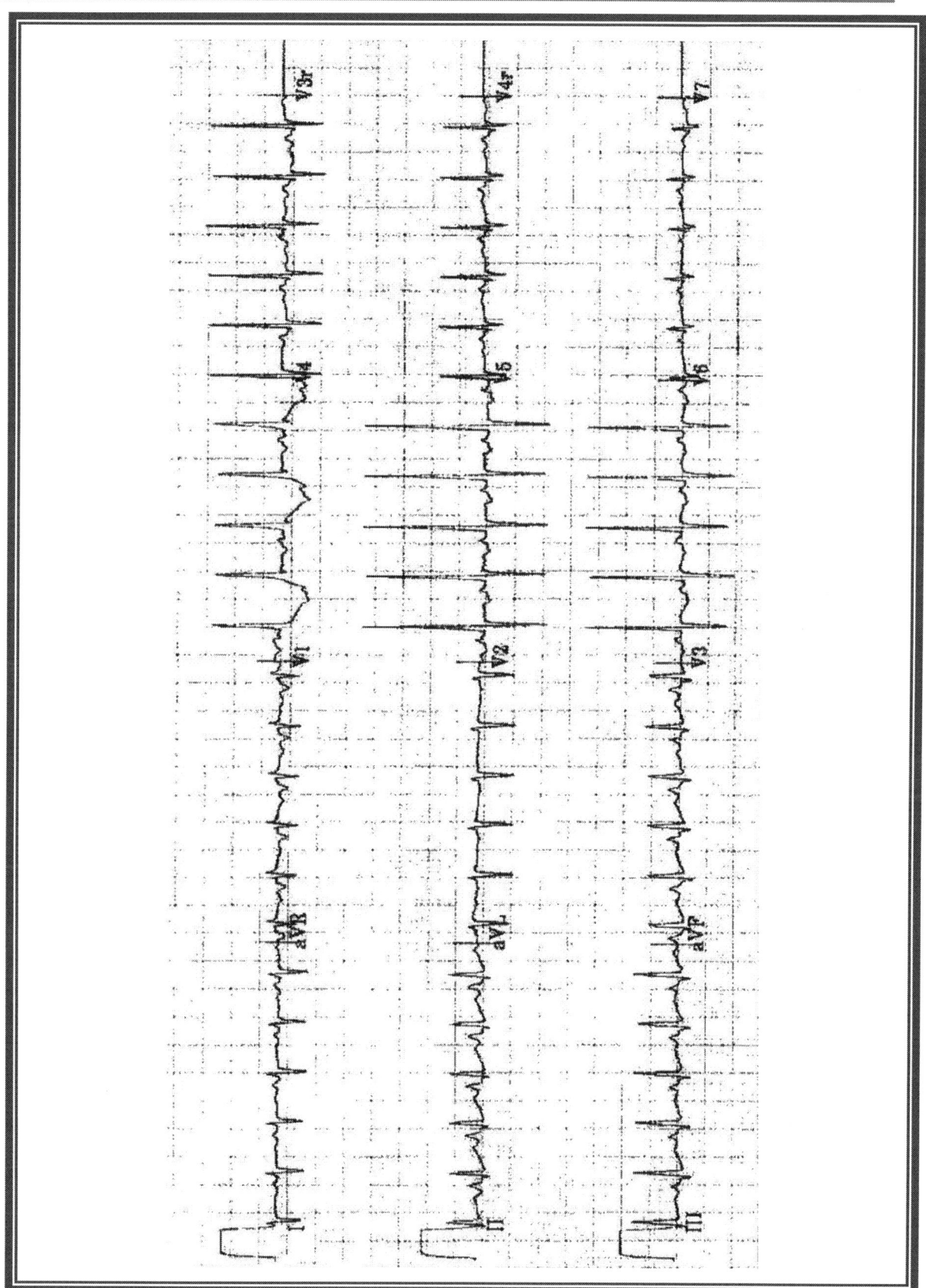

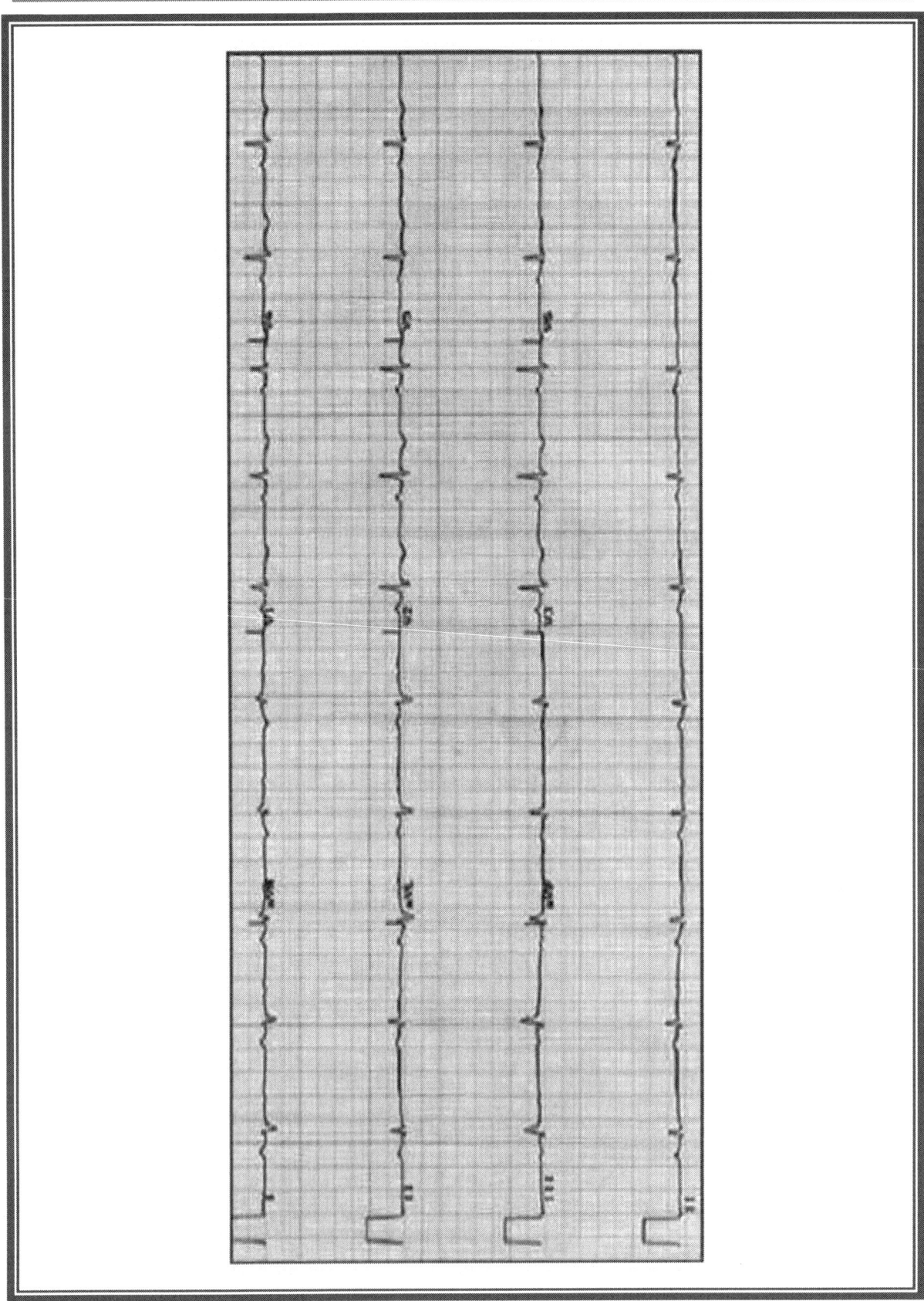

WRITE THE DIAGNOSIS OF THE PREVIOUS EKG'S:

1. _____

2. _____

3. _____

4. _____

5. _____

6. _____

7. _____

8. _____

9. _____

10. _____

11. _____

12. _____

13. _____

14. _____

15. _____

16. _____

17. _____

18. _____

19. _____

20. _____

21. _____

22. _____

23. _____

24. _____

25. _____

WRITE THE DIAGNOSIS OF THE PREVIOUS EKG'S:

26. _____

27. _____

28. _____

29. _____

30. _____

31. _____

32. _____

33. _____

34. _____

35. _____

36. _____

37. _____

38. _____

CHECK OUT:

12 Lead EKG In About an Hour!

*AVAILABLE BOTH PAPERBACK AND ELECTRONIC.

Printed in Great Britain
by Amazon

57306628R00061